RESTORATIVE
YOGA
for beginners

RESTORATIVE YOGA *for beginners*

GENTLE POSES FOR RELAXATION AND HEALING

JULIA CLARKE

ROCKRIDGE
PRESS

First Rockridge Press trade paperback edition 2019

Rockridge Press and the Rockridge Press logo are trademarks or registered trademarks of Callisto Media Inc. and/or its affiliates in the United States and other countries and may not be used without written permission.

For general information on our other products and services, please contact our Customer Care Department within the United States at (866) 744-2665, or outside the United States at (510) 253-0500.

Paperback ISBN: 978-1-64611-184-8 | eBook ISBN: 978-1-64611-185-5

Manufactured in the United States of America

Interior and Cover Designer: Lindsey Dekker
Art Producer: Michael Hardgrove
Editor: Sean Newcott
Production Editor: Jenna Dutton
Production Manager: Holly Haydash
Illustrations: Christy Ni
Author photo courtesy of © Kate Broussard Photography

10 9 8 7 6 5 4 3 2 1

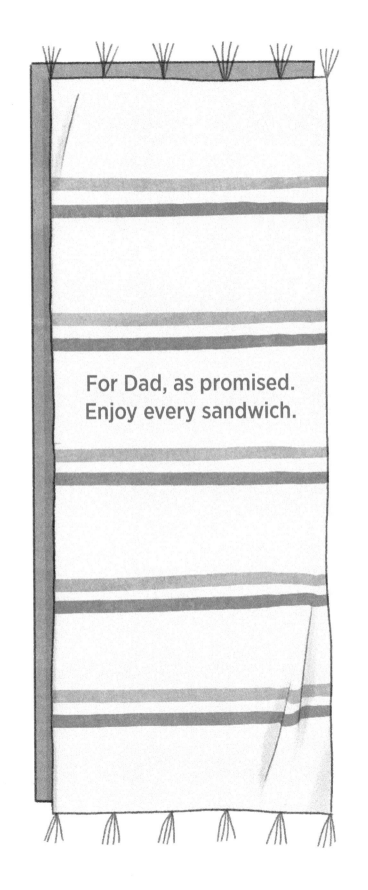

For Dad, as promised.
Enjoy every sandwich.

Contents

Introduction

The practice of restorative yoga has resulted in life-changing results for many of my students. Take Marissa, for example. With her foot firmly on the gas pedal since college, any hope of deep sleep was thwarted by hectic, caffeine-fueled days juggling career, marriage, and children. Her only "relaxation" came when she collapsed onto the couch at the end of the night with a glass of wine and a sleeping pill to help her power down for what typically amounted to a restless night.

Shortly after her 56th birthday, she and her family took their annual ski trip to Colorado. Unable to ignore the aches, pains, and exhaustion she'd long been experiencing, Marissa skipped a day of racing her young grandkids down the slopes and stepped into her first restorative yoga class with me. Bracing herself for an intimidating physical challenge she'd come to equate with yoga, she was surprised to start class lying down, supported by soft blankets and pillows. Twenty minutes in, she had drifted off into a state of deep relaxation. Her mind did an extraordinary thing—it quieted down. Years of tension began to melt from her muscles. That night, she slept soundly and woke the next day feeling more recharged and hopeful than she had in years. Upon returning home, she continued a regular restorative yoga practice, and when I saw her back in Vail the following winter, she was 20 pounds lighter, sleeping again, and feeling happier. She attributed her transformation to her yoga practice.

Instead of moving through challenging standing poses, the therapeutic practice of restorative yoga uses supported positions to invoke deep relaxation to settle your mind and harmonize your physiology. It can relieve stress and pain and improve emotional well-being. I've seen it equally benefit teenagers and seniors, athletes and pregnant women, people dealing with chronic illness and those recovering from surgery.

After years of dedicating myself to a very active yoga practice, I discovered restorative yoga when I was healing from injuries sustained in a serious bike accident. After my first class, I knew I had found something that could unlock years of stress for me and my students. What's more, unlike the energetic vinyasa yoga classes I was already teaching, restorative yoga was an accessible practice that absolutely anyone can do. I signed up for teacher training and began studying with a group of incredible women who credited the practice with helping them overcome such challenges as crippling anxiety, depression, breast cancer, and lupus. Six months later—despite feeling convinced that persuading mountain athletes to relax would be an uphill battle—my first restorative yoga class sold out.

Today, as a teacher, business owner, and Ayurvedic practitioner, restorative yoga is something I rely on to help sustain my joy for life, my passion for teaching, and to nourish my energy and creativity. Through my own teacher trainings, it is my great honor to help others discover restorative yoga's benefits as well.

I hope this book will convince you of the merits of restorative yoga, but also of your ability to enjoy these benefits—regardless of who you are. Whether old or young, experienced or beginner, injured or sick, or just seeking more from your practice, restorative yoga is for you.

How to Use This Book

This book contains everything you need to know to start your restorative yoga practice from scratch, deepen your existing practice, or support your students if you are a teacher. Its contents come from my own experience and passion for getting everybody to relax more.

Part I describes restorative yoga—what it is, where it comes from, and how it works on your nervous system to facilitate the elusive state of deep relaxation. We'll discuss its potential benefits and cover practical details such as what to wear when you're practicing, what props you'll need (as well as how to make your own props with what you already have at home), and, finally, how to create a lasting habit out of your practice.

Part II contains a detailed and illustrated guide to the gentle, relaxing poses at the heart of restorative yoga. Rest assured, these are poses anyone can do. You will also find 19 sequences you can follow at home for a profoundly rejuvenating experience and tips for creating your own sequences. One thing I have learned in my years of teaching and practicing restorative yoga is that the less you have to think about it, the more effective it is at soothing your nervous system. So, for each pose, I explain how it acts upon your body, how much time to spend in it, what props are needed, the precautions to take, and the benefits.

One thing that sets restorative yoga apart from most styles of yoga is that you are not seeking to create any intense physical sensation, such as a deep stretch. Modern biomechanics suggest that the stretch sensation is actually your nervous system detecting an unfamiliar range of motion and responding with a fight-or-flight mechanism of contraction to guard your body against a perceived threat. In this practice, you focus on cultivating the nervous system's relaxation response, in which your muscles are supported and the sensation is one of gentle opening— these poses should be very comfortable and soothing. (Note that if you experience pain, you should modify the pose or try a different pose.)

Although I have outlined poses to help with pain, stress relief, and pregnancy, please remember this book and the practice of restorative yoga are not intended to act as a substitute for professional medical care. Consult your doctor regarding important medical decisions, but I encourage you to consider this book as a partner on your journey toward better health.

Finally, I want to assure you that no matter where you are in life, I believe this book can set you on a course toward a healthier, happier life with less pain and less stress. This, in turn, can help you generate a more optimistic outlook, improve your relationships, and help you create the fulfilling life you desire and deserve. Let's dive in.

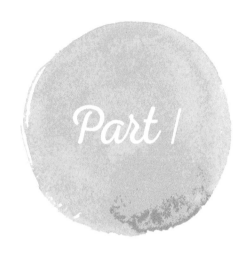

Part I

All About Restorative Yoga

CHAPTER 1

Restorative Yoga Basics

Restorative yoga is a practice of conscious relaxation, using props in every posture to support your muscles in gentle, comfortable positions. It is distinctly devoid of poses like Downward Facing Dog and Cobra that are the keystones of other popular styles. In fact, the mainstay of a restorative yoga practice is Basic Relaxation Pose (page 26), essentially a supported Corpse Pose (*Savasana*), which you hold for up to 30 minutes at a time. Other poses include gentle reclining backbends, supine twists, and supported forward folds and hip openers. The poses are held for anywhere from 3 to 30 minutes, giving your body plenty of time to relax, so that your mind can enter a quiet, meditative state.

The Origins of Restorative Yoga

Restorative yoga is a style of hatha yoga, which historians believe emerged in 10th-century India. It encompasses all practices that use postures to target your physical body as a means to access and transform the inner landscape of energy, mind, and emotions. Meaning "sun-moon," hatha yoga aims to balance passive "lunar" energy with active "solar" energy, or yin (lunar) with yang (solar) in traditional Chinese medicine terms. As such, you can view restorative yoga as a lunar practice using relaxation to balance the excessive action of modern life.

Its roots lie with B. K. S. Iyengar, a pioneer in using props such as blankets, blocks, and straps to avoid straining in poses. His student Judith Hanson Lasater became instrumental in popularizing restorative yoga in the United States beginning in the 1970s. She created thoughtful sequences for pregnancy, back pain, headaches, and insomnia outlined in her book *Relax and Renew*. My restorative yoga teacher, Shannon Paige, studied with Lasater after she found the practice to be vital during her recovery from cancer.

And although historically it has not enjoyed the same popularity as movement-based styles such as Ashtanga and vinyasa yoga, restorative yoga is gaining momentum. An encouraging 2018 study conducted by the website DOYOUYOGA found restorative yoga to be the third most practiced style of yoga. Its growth has no doubt been fueled by our collective awareness of the documented toxic effects of chronic stress and increasing focus on therapeutic wellness practices. Studies increasingly point to the efficacy of yoga, meditation, and relaxation for stress reduction. With its effectiveness and accessibility, restorative yoga has the potential to become a major player in the field of stress management in years to come.

What Makes Restorative Yoga Different?

Many turn to yoga for stress relief only to find themselves gasping for air in fast-paced, competitive classes and forcing their bodies into impossible shapes. In restorative yoga, deep relaxation, supported postures, gentle breathing, and meditation work together to ease stress by trading the push of productivity for the gifts of receptivity.

Ours is a world that values action and rewards results. You're told by the media that you're not enough and you don't have enough and that the solution is to do more and accumulate more. The concepts of rest and receptivity are neither prized nor commonly practiced, and the resulting epidemic of stress is feeding that of chronic disease as we adapt to the mounting pressures of modern life.

Imagine this: After another stressful, relentless, white-knuckle day at work you enter a quiet, softly lit room. On your yoga mat are blankets and cushions. You lie down, supported, and feel your body finally relaxing. You exhale. You feel a deep, inner stillness: a pause between breaths where you feel steady and free. Liberated from the confines of worry, the tidal wave of thoughts subsides. The spinning stops. After a few poses, you emerge renewed. That night, you sleep deeply, and, in the morning, you feel a little less stressed by the unending flow of email, traffic, and demands.

This is the power of restorative yoga. Instead of poses like headstand and plank that strengthen your muscles against gravity, you find postures that elicit total mind-body relaxation. The ongoing self-analysis of critical thinking surrenders to heart-centered self-compassion and nonjudgment where true healing can begin.

Restorative yoga is based on these principles:

- A focus on opening and relaxation, not strength or flexibility
- Poses are held for up to 30 minutes, giving you time to relax completely
- The practice uses props in every pose to facilitate relaxation states that can otherwise be elusive
- The poses are simple and gentle, making it appropriate for everyone
- Each practice consists of only a handful of postures
- It promotes states of peaceful contemplation, abundance, and well-being

Other Styles of Yoga

Ashtanga yoga: Developed by Sri K. Pattabhi Jois, this dynamic, vigorous yoga practice syncs movement with breath. Ashtanga yoga consists of six increasingly advanced sequences that include sun salutations, standing poses, arm balances, and deep backbends.

Bikram yoga: Created by Bikram Choudhury, this style of hot yoga features 26 postures and two breathing exercises practiced in a room heated to somewhere between 95°F and 108°F.

Iyengar yoga: Named after its founder, B. K. S. Iyengar, this practice emphasizes precision in alignment within postures and heavily features the use of props.

Kundalini yoga: Brought to the West by Yogi Bhajan, kundalini yoga centers on dynamic and forceful movements and breath work with chanting and meditation to move subtle energy, known as "kundalini energy."

Vinyasa flow: Meaning "to place in a special way," this creative and dynamic practice emerged in Southern California from students of Ashtanga yoga. Although the term may be used to describe a wide range of styles from Shiva Rea's prana flow to power yoga, it denotes a flowing practice in which breath and movement are thoughtfully aligned.

Yin yoga: Based on Paulie Zink's Taoist yoga and developed by Paul Grilley and Sarah Powers, yin yoga features long holds in deep stretches to stress the body's connective tissues and uses the meridians of traditional Chinese medicine as a guide. The postures are typically seated or reclining. Although physically distinct from restorative yoga, yin yoga is by far the most energetically similar style of yoga to restorative.

"Anthropologists tell us the body that experiences stress has not changed much over the millions of years of being human. Our ancestors had the same anatomical and physiological characteristics as we who drive freeways and communicate via the information superhighway. We have an ancient body subjected to a modern problem: living with chronic stress." —Judith Hanson Lasater

The Benefits of Restorative Yoga

Restorative yoga has the power to drastically improve the quality of your life and, subsequently, the lives of those around you. What's more, this isn't a "VIP Only" area—you can reap these benefits the moment you start practicing, regardless of your experience level.

Stress management. Relaxation has been shown to reduce stress hormones, such as cortisol and adrenaline. The Mayo Clinic lists many ways relaxation can help physiologically reduce stress, including slowing heart rate, lowering blood pressure, improving concentration and mood, improving sleep quality, reducing fatigue, diminishing feelings of anger and frustration, and boosting problem-solving abilities.

Healthier respiration. Shallow breathing is common in our computer-driven society, and it can provoke anxiety, back pain, brain fog, and poor digestion. The book *Breath in Action* asserts that simply paying more attention to your breath can help. In restorative yoga you soften the respiration muscles through comfortable postures, then bring awareness to your breath and employ gentle breathing practices.

Improved digestion. When stress triggers the fight-or-flight response, the sympathetic nervous system interferes with the enteric nervous system's ability to digest food. Restorative yoga encourages the positive "rest and digest" function of the parasympathetic nervous system. A Harvard Health Publishing article correlated relaxation therapies, like progressive muscle relaxation and visualization, with gastrointestinal relief.

Pain relief. Causes of pain include stress, poor posture, inadequate breathing, and inflammation, all of which restorative yoga addresses. An article published in the *International Journal of Yoga* cited a significant reduction in chronic and acute pain when relaxation techniques were applied.

Weight loss. A Yale study links high secretion of the stress hormone cortisol with an increase in abdominal fat. Because stress is the primary factor in its development, this type of fat is better targeted with relaxation than strenuous exercise.

Emotional well-being. Restorative yoga fosters states of peace, joy, and compassion. Also, by receiving support and bringing your awareness to the unlimited supply of breath available to you, you shift your perspective from scarcity to abundance.

Who Can Do Restorative Yoga?

Everyone can benefit from restorative yoga—these days we all need to reduce our stress levels. Fortunately, it's such an accessible practice literally anyone can do it, regardless of conditioning, age, or injuries. Take my former student Jeremy, for example. When we met, Jeremy, a lifelong runner, had recently undergone a hip replacement surgery. He had never stretched a day in his life and now, in his late 60s, he was experiencing pain and significant restriction in his range of motion. He was ready to invite more balance into his life, but the thought of stepping into a traditional yoga class terrified him.

With encouragement from his friends and family, he finally agreed to try restorative yoga. Much to his amazement, he was able to move through an entire sequence, simply adding more blankets for support whenever he felt any discomfort. As time went by, his pain subsided and his mobility improved.

Another student, Carla, came to me seeking stress relief during a "surprise" pregnancy. She already had three young children at home and was more than a little overwhelmed at the prospect of welcoming another. Using pregnancy modifications, restorative yoga proved ideal for her during those stressful times and allowed her, as the primary caregiver in her family, to feel cared for and nurtured.

Restorative yoga can benefit anyone, but stories like these show its accessibility makes it particularly ideal for:

- Anyone with extreme stress
- Beginners
- People dealing with illness
- People with disabilities
- People with injuries
- Pregnant women
- Seniors

How It Works

Contemporary yoga practices may look like an exercise regime but, at its core, yoga is a spiritual discipline. Yoga uses many tools to reunite your body with your mind and consciousness and regain mastery over your thoughts and actions to alleviate suffering. Modern science helps you understand the physical benefits of restorative yoga, and yoga philosophy informs its spiritual power.

A sixth-century BCE yoga text, the *Taittiriya Upanishad*, outlines five layers to human existence, called *koshas*, which offer an insightful map to help you navigate the spiritual journey you take in restorative yoga. These five layers comprise the physical body, energy/breath, mind/emotions, intellect, and the blissful layer of consciousness where you are unburdened by body, emotions, or thoughts. Pain or tension in one layer will affect all others, and restorative yoga is a pathway to harmonizing all five.

Restorative yoga first supports your body, easing physical tension. This helps restore the natural, easy breath you enjoyed as an infant. When your breath and body soften, your mind can open to what *is* happening (you are relaxing, supported, and safe), releasing what it's worried *might* happen. When your mind quiets down, your discerning intellect kicks in, retaking control over the direction of your mind. The contraction of worry and lack gives way to spacious feelings of abundance and ease. Arriving at this sweet spot, known as the bliss layer, is the core journey in restorative yoga. The reintegration of physical and subtle body at the heart of yoga is believed to reduce suffering and support your evolution.

The Five Koshas

Annamaya Kosha
physical body

Pranamaya Kosha
vital energy, breath, auras, chakras

Manomaya Kosha
mind, perceptual organization, habits, language, emotions

Vijnanamaya Kosha
intellect, wisdom, discernment, critical thinking, inner witness

Anandamaya Kosha
bliss, the totality of human potential, inner harmony, peace, intuition, self-confidence, equanimity, well-being

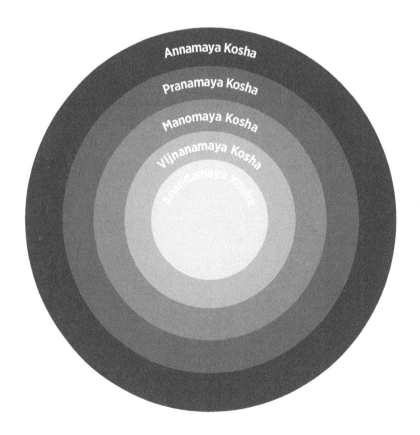

The Medical View

Understanding the alchemy of stress is key to the medical explanation for how restorative yoga works. *Psychology Today* called the elevated levels of cortisol that stress provokes "public enemy number one," with symptoms including poor memory, low immunity, weight gain, and hypertension.

The fight-or-flight response comes with cases of extreme stress, like when you hear the screech of tires at a busy intersection or get into an argument. It's a holdover from your ancestors, whose nervous systems developed an emergency response system for when they encountered a predator. The perception of threat elevates cortisol production, the nervous system shuts down all "unnecessary" systems, such as rational thinking and digestion, and floods the body with glucose, narrowing the arteries, accelerating the breath rate, and elevating the heart rate to prepare for combat.

Today, the chances of being eaten by a hungry lion while foraging for food at the grocery store are decidedly low, but anything from major life changes to the posture and shallow breathing that come with slouching at a computer for long periods can incite this ancient response. That's right: stress can be triggered by even the most mundane aspects of modern life, like sitting. A University of Auckland study identified a direct correlation between modern posture and increasing emotional stress, and it may all come down to how our posture affects our breath. Right now, hunch over and observe how you feel. Do you feel joyful or depressed? Can you breathe deeply? Now stand up, throw your arms out wide, and smile. How does this feel in comparison? You know that when you're anxious you can't breathe, but did you know that when you don't breathe properly, you may be making yourself anxious? The very posture you spend the most time in may be the most harmful one for our physical and emotional health.

By simply taking the first step of lying down, relaxing, and breathing softly in restorative yoga, you activate the relaxation response of your parasympathetic nervous system and begin to reverse the harmful effects of stress.

CHAPTER 2

What to Know Before You Begin

Now that we've looked at how restorative yoga can help you establish more balance in your life, it's time to get down to the nuts and bolts of what you'll need to begin your practice. This chapter covers everything from how much time you'll need and how to create a supportive space for your practice to what to wear and what props you'll need so you feel prepared to successfully begin your restorative yoga practice at home— and even feel comfortable taking public classes.

What You'll Need

The following are the essential items for your restorative yoga toolkit so you can get started straightaway. As you'll see, there's no need to invest a stack of money to acquire new props and toys for this practice; in fact, you'll likely find you already have everything you need at home.

Time

Time is probably the most precious and limited commodity you have, so rest assured you may not need to set aside as much of it as you think to benefit from the practice. Any pose in this book may be held for as few as 3 minutes, though some days your practice might mean you spend 20 minutes in Basic Relaxation Pose (page 26). When you only have 5 minutes and you've been on your feet all day, spend them in Legs Up the Wall (page 62). When you have more time, follow a full sequence for sustained relaxation. You can practice restorative yoga at any time of the day when it works for your schedule.

A full yoga sequence leaves you feeling completely replenished for hours, or even days, so a good goal is to aim for an hour-long practice once or twice a week, then top up with short mini-sequences as you have time. And don't worry—there's no such thing as doing too much restorative yoga!

Space

The next thing to consider is space. Like time, you really don't need much of it. You can set aside an entire room or just one corner of a room. Unroll your yoga mat and lie on it to make sure you have enough room to stretch your arms up overhead and roll over onto one side without bumping into anything.

It's helpful to keep the space you practice in clean and tidy so you're not distracted by things you feel you need to clean up and organize. It should be quiet, warm enough to stay comfortable, and somewhere your kids and pets won't start climbing all over you the moment you lie down. Dim the lights and turn off all electronics to avoid disruptions. Feel free to set a relaxing tone with essential oils, candles, or soothing music.

If you're planning to practice at work, find the quietest, most distraction-free space available; ideally an office or room with a door you can close for privacy.

There's no special uniform or new wardrobe items you need to purchase to practice restorative yoga. You simply want to be comfortable and warm enough, as your body temperature tends to drop by a degree or two when you're resting. I encourage my students to dress in soft, loose, comfortable layers, and yes, that includes pajamas. As a general rule of thumb, wear loose-fitting pants, socks, and long sleeves that can be removed if you get too warm. Avoid tight-fitting clothing that restricts movement or breathing, itchy fabrics, and annoying zippers and fasteners. Comfort is the name of the game.

Props

An essential component of any restorative yoga practice, props serve the important role of supporting you so your muscles can relax completely. However, you don't have to purchase lots of expensive new yoga props to begin. In fact, you can easily use items you have around the house. In this section, you'll see that props are divided into "essential" items that you likely already have, and "nice-to-have" props that you may choose to buy. (See page 155 for recommendations on where to buy props.) Here, you'll learn how to fold blankets and create your own props.

Essential Props

This is a list of items you likely have around the house. Remember, you can do an entire restorative yoga practice with only these props.

- Yoga mat and a blanket to lie on (or 2 blankets)
- Blanket to cover yourself
- 1 to 3 additional blankets (or large bath towels) to build bolsters
- 2 yoga blocks (or large hardcover books)
- 1 or 2 bulky pillows from your bed (or cushions from your couch)
- Medium bath towel you can use as a pillow with neck support
- Small towel or washcloth to cover your eyes
- Chair without wheels (optional; for use with chair poses)

If you're interested in acquiring some specialized restorative yoga props, here's a list of items that would be a great place to start.

- 1 or 2 rectangular bolsters (approximate dimensions: 25" L x 6" H x 12" W)
- 1 round bolster (approximate dimensions: 28" x 10")
- 1 pranayama bolster (this can be used in place of a blanket roll in many postures; approximate dimensions: 25" L x 6" H x 3" W)
- 2 to 4 yoga blankets or traditional Mexican blankets (approximate dimensions 73" x 48")
- Eye pillow
- Neck pillow
- Yoga sandbag (approximately 7 to 10 pounds, these can be placed on any body part to add weight and augment the sensation of grounding and relaxation)
- Yoga strap

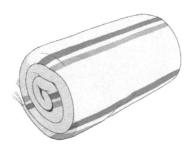

These are the four basic blanket folds for your restorative yoga practice:

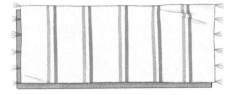

Half-fold blanket

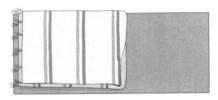

Quarter-fold blanket

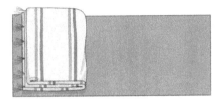

Square eighth-fold blanket

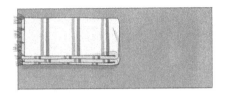

Long eighth-fold blanket

Using these, you can easily make the following props:

- **Make your own bolster.** Take 2 half-fold blankets, lay one on top of the other, and roll them up starting at the narrow end. To make a larger bolster, use 3 blankets.

- **Make your own blanket roll.** Take one quarter-fold blanket and roll it up along the long edge to make a long, thin tube.

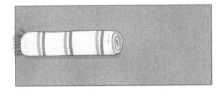

- **Make your own neck pillow.** Take one eighth-fold blanket and place it under your head, then roll up the end closest to your neck until it fills the gap between the back of your neck and the blanket.

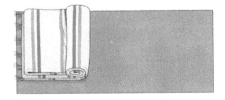

Making Progress

The beauty of restorative yoga is that it's not about progressing to more advanced postures but becoming more fluent in the language of relaxation. In fact, although at first you may be curious about trying all the poses in this book, over time you will come to learn what is most effective for your body and you may find you experience deep relaxation practicing just a few poses. To that end, forgo poses that don't feel relaxing to you—that's okay.

If you're entering into this practice with injuries, please follow the instructions to use more or less support as needed so you don't worsen your symptoms. There's no benefit to pushing through pain or discomfort here. Remember, the journey is the practice; we're not trying to get to a particular destination. This is a practice of finding what works for you and doing it until it becomes a healthy habit.

Taking Classes

Today there are many restorative yoga classes offered from basic sequences to specialized classes that use music, aromatherapy, Reiki, and other complementary practices. If you're curious about taking restorative yoga classes, they can be a great way to supplement your home practice. Once you feel comfortable, you might find that taking a class allows you to feel even more supported and relaxed as the teacher handles all the planning. A good teacher may even offer guided visualizations, meditations, and breath work to enhance your journey.

Before taking a class, reach out to the studio or gym to ensure that the class is a true restorative yoga class, as some may actually be a slow-flow class and an entirely different experience. Some teachers offer hands-on assists, so if you are not comfortable with this, let them know in advance.

A Note to Teachers

- As a teacher, you may use this book for your own personal growth or to help you plan your own restorative yoga class sequences. If you work with older students or those dealing with injuries or illnesses, this practice can be an extremely powerful addition to your class roster, helping you connect with your students and offering them a pathway to healing.
- If you think your community might be hesitant to try restorative yoga, adding one to three restorative poses at the end of a more physically challenging practice can be an effective way to introduce your students to the benefits without them having to commit to a full hour. I suggest beginning with Basic Relaxation Pose (page 26), Heart Pose (page 34), and Supported Child's Pose (page 38).
- You may have to get creative if your studio or gym lacks props, but remember that yoga mats can be rolled up to create bolsters and towels can be used as blankets and pillows.
- Finally, restorative yoga is extremely popular when offered as a special class or workshop. Because your students spend so much time in each pose, this presents a great opportunity for you to guide a special theme (like "writing" a story of self-compassion to replace a narrative of self-doubt with positive intentions), or to weave in your knowledge of subjects such as yoga mythology or the chakras.

Forming a Habit

Although there are no official guidelines for how often you should practice, studies suggest that the more regularly you practice yoga and meditation, the greater the benefits. However, forming new, healthy habits can be challenging: You're busy and, likely, hard-wired toward instant gratification—and healthy habits don't always deliver immediate results. For help with overcoming this hurdle, we can turn to James Clear, author of *Atomic Habits*, and these five helpful tips of his:

1. **Start small.** Practice for 20 minutes in Basic Relaxation Pose (page 26) once a week.
2. **Increase slowly.** After a couple of weeks, progress to 30 minutes, adding another posture or two.
3. **Break it up.** As the time increases it's helpful to break it up into chunks. Once you hit 60 minutes, split the time into two 30-minute practices.
4. **Plan for failure.** You will miss a practice and, when you do, just return to it as quickly as possible. Missing a practice won't detract from your overall progress.
5. **Practice patience.** Like any new habit, restorative yoga gets easier the more you do it.

Dos and Don'ts

Keep these basic tips in mind to keep your practice on the right path.

Do:

Designate a self-care day. If you feel overwhelmed with incorporating another thing into your weekly routine, set aside one morning or one evening a week to enjoy all your self-care rituals.

Reward yourself. A study from Iowa State University suggests that adding a motivating reward, such as a bite of chocolate, after your practice is key to making your habit stick.

Identify barriers to your success. It's helpful to understand why you're struggling with consistency. Is it a lack of time? Start with 10 minutes. An issue with space? Create a designated restorative yoga area at home. The absence of motivation? Invite a friend to come to a class with you.

Set unrealistic goals. If you've never done yoga before, there's no need to make a goal to practice for an hour a day. You may get busy and miss a day of practice and feel like you've failed yourself. Start small.

Lose yourself in self-doubt. It's normal to feel daunted by new things. Just remember, everyone can lie down and that's precisely where we start. Next, you can focus on becoming the pilot of your mind rather than the passenger.

Worry that you're being selfish. Self-care can be unfamiliar terrain and, sometimes, you can mistake it for self-indulgence. But without it you grow depleted, short-tempered, and impatient with others. Think of restorative yoga as the gift you give to everyone you meet.

Did you know the brain waves you experience in conscious relaxation are different from sleep?

Theta brain waves are associated with daydreaming and REM sleep during which we experience rapid eye movement and dreams that can trigger stress. Delta brain waves are associated with deep, dreamless sleep. In practices such as restorative yoga, you experience alpha brain waves, which are associated with deep relaxation and are believed to serve as a bridge between conscious thinking and the subconscious mind.

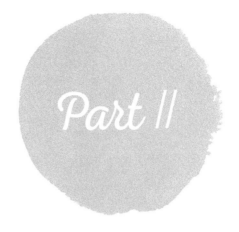

Poses and Sequences

The next four chapters describe in detail the poses of restorative yoga, how to do them, and the props you'll need, followed by chapters providing sequences for practice as well as breathing exercises and meditations you may want to incorporate into your practice.

Please note that for each pose, in addition to the props listed, you'll of course need your yoga mat. I also recommend laying a half-fold blanket over your mat for added comfort and keeping another blanket nearby to cover yourself in case you need a little extra warmth. In any of the reclining postures, you may cover your eyes with an eye pillow or small washcloth to help you relax more deeply.

CHAPTER 3

Poses: The Basics

The next four chapters describe in detail the poses of restorative yoga, how to do them, and the props you'll need, followed by chapters providing sequences for practice as well as breathing exercises and meditations you may want to incorporate into your practice. Please note that for each pose, in addition to the props listed, you'll of course need your yoga mat. I also recommend laying a half-fold blanket over your mat for added comfort and keeping another blanket nearby to cover yourself in case you need a little extra warmth. In any of the reclining postures, you may cover your eyes with an eye pillow or small washcloth to help you relax more deeply.

Basic Relaxation Pose

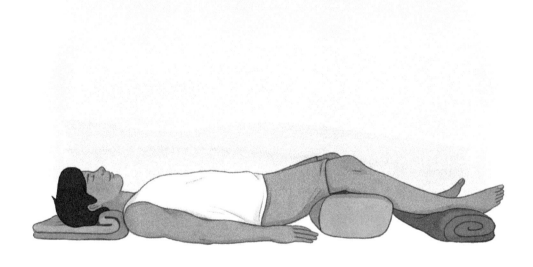

PROPS

Bolster (or 2 rolled
blankets or
a large pillow)

Blanket roll

Square eighth-fold
blanket (or neck pillow)

- If you are pregnant, substitute Pregnant Goddess (page 86) or Side Lying Pose (page 88).
- If you experience lower back or knee pain, place two blocks under your bolster or roll up three blankets to make a bigger bolster.

BENEFITS

- Maintains and supports the natural curves of your spine.
- Softens your psoas, the deep hip flexor muscles that can become chronically contracted if you spend extended periods sitting, and diaphragm muscle to support a natural, easy breath.
- Relaxes your whole body to aid in stress reduction, slows heart rate, and lowers blood pressure.
- Helps relieve lower back pain.
- Encourages feelings of grounding, belonging, and peace.

TIP

Adding weight can help make this pose feel even more grounding. Place a heavy folded blanket or yoga sandbag on your chest or across your lap to help you relax more deeply.

INSTRUCTIONS

1. From a sitting position, draw your knees over the bolster and rest your ankles on the blanket roll.
2. Lie back and rest your head on the eighth-fold blanket. Roll up the edge of the blanket so it supports the curve of your neck without forcing your chin toward your chest.
3. Cover yourself with a blanket, cover your eyes, and release your arms alongside your body.
4. Remain in Basic Relaxation Pose for up to 30 minutes. To exit, draw your knees in toward your chest, roll to one side, and press yourself up to a sitting position.

Simple Supported Side Bend

3 to 5 minutes per side

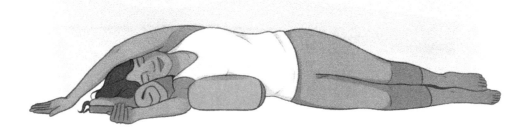

PROPS

Bolster (or 2 rolled blankets or a large pillow)

Square eighth-fold blanket

- If you have a spinal injury, replace the bolster with one or two stacked long eighth-fold blankets to reduce the curve in your spine.

BENEFITS

- Gently stretches your obliques, latissimus dorsi, and intercostal muscles.
- Gently decompresses your spine.
- Invites your breath to deepen.
- Supports and maintains your spine in normal, healthy lateral flexion.
- Helps relieve lower back pain.
- Encourages a feeling of flexibility.

TIP

Place a blanket or pillow between your knees for more support or to relieve discomfort in your knees or hips.

INSTRUCTIONS

1. Sit on your right hip with your knees bent and feet tucked behind you and bring the long edge of the bolster up against your right thigh.
2. Roll up the blanket and place it on the other side of the bolster with a small gap in between.
3. Lay your right side over the bolster, placing your right shoulder in the gap between the bolster and the blanket. Release your right arm out in front of you and rest your head on the blanket.
4. Rest your left arm on your side, or draw it up alongside your left ear for a little more length.
5. Remain in the side bend for 3 to 5 minutes. To exit, place your left hand onto the bolster and press yourself up. Leave the props as they are and turn yourself around to sitting on your left hip to repeat the pose on the other side.

Grounding Spinal Twist

Twist • 3 to 5 minutes per side

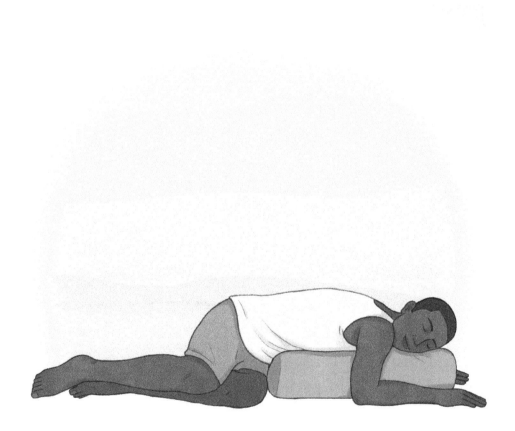

Bolster (or 2 rolled blankets or a large pillow)

- If spinal rotation is contraindicated for you (in the case of spinal injury or pregnancy), skip this pose.

BENEFITS

- Supports and maintains your spine in normal, healthy rotation.
- Gently decompresses your spine.
- Gently stretches your lumbar muscles.
- Helps relieve back pain.
- Invites feelings of connection and stability.

TIP

It's common to try to support yourself with your arms in this pose, so make sure to take your elbows a little wider and relax, letting the bolster do the work for you.

INSTRUCTIONS

1. Sit on your right hip with your knees bent and your feet tucked in behind you and bring the narrow end of the bolster up against your right hip.
2. Place your hands on either side of the bolster. Sit up tall and turn your navel and heart toward the bolster. Slowly lower your torso down and place either cheek on the bolster.
3. Remain in the twist for 3 to 5 minutes. To exit, place your hands on either side of the bolster and press yourself up. Leave the bolster where it is and turn yourself around to sitting on your left hip to repeat the pose on the other side.

Spine Lengthening Pose

Backbend • 5 to 10 minutes

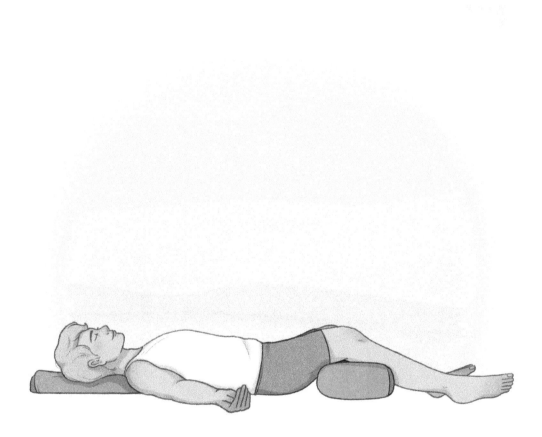

PROPS

Bolster (or 2 rolled blankets or a large pillow)

Blanket roll

- If you are pregnant, substitute Pregnant Goddess Pose (page 86) or Supported Heart Pose with Legs Over a Bolster (page 66).

BENEFITS

- Gently decompresses your spine.
- Supports and maintains your spine in normal, healthy extension.
- Gently stretches your chest and shoulders.
- Reverses the effects of long periods spent sitting and slouching.
- Invites your breath to deepen.
- Encourages feelings of spaciousness and receptivity.

TIP

A common error is to sit on the blanket roll before lying down and miss out on the spinal massage in this pose. Make sure your hips are between the bolster and blanket roll before you lie down to create length.

INSTRUCTIONS

1. From a sitting position, draw your knees over the bolster and position the end of the blanket roll at the base of your spine.
2. Use your arms for support and lie back so the blanket roll runs along the length of your spine and supports your head.
3. Release your arms alongside you with your palms facing up and relax.
4. Remain in Spine Lengthening Pose for 5 to 10 minutes. To exit, draw your knees in toward your chest, roll to one side, and press yourself up to a sitting position.

Heart Pose

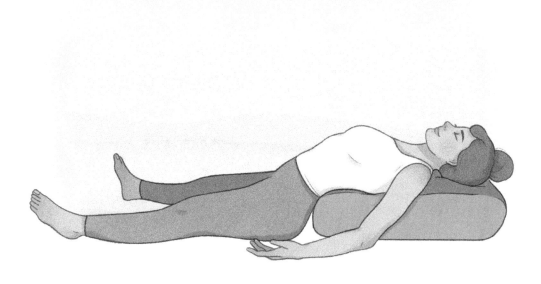

PROPS

Bolster (or 2 rolled blankets or a large pillow)

- If you are pregnant, substitute Pregnant Goddess Pose (page 86).
- If you suffer from lower back pain or sensitivity, substitute Supported Heart Pose with Legs Over a Bolster (page 66).

BENEFITS

- Gently decompresses your spine.
- Gently stretches your chest, shoulders, and abdomen.
- Reverses the effects of long periods spent sitting and slouching.
- Invites your breath to deepen.
- Naturally boosts your energy and supports feelings of joy and abundance.

TIP

If the bolster feels too high for your spine in this position and the sensation is too intense, move your hips away from the bolster slightly to create some space and lessen the curve in your spine.

INSTRUCTIONS

1. From a sitting position, extend your legs out in front of you and bring the narrow end of the bolster up to the base of your spine. Using your arms for support, relax your abdominal muscles and lie back onto the bolster.
2. Remain in Heart Pose for 5 to 10 minutes. To exit, bend your knees, roll to one side, and press yourself up to a sitting position.

Supported Forward Fold

Forward Bend • 5 to 8 minutes

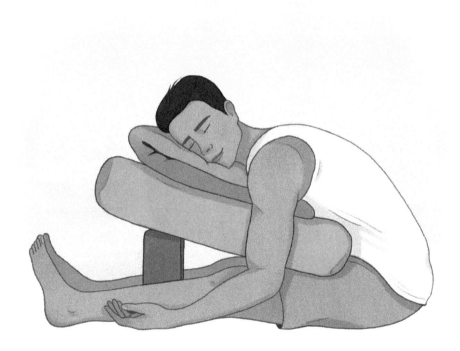

PROPS

Bolster (or 2 rolled blankets or a large pillow)	Block (or large hardcover book)	Square eighth-fold blanket

- If forward bending is contraindicated for your spine, substitute Legs Up the Wall (page 62) or Head to Bolster Pose (page 76).

BENEFITS

- Supports and maintains your spine in normal, healthy flexion.
- Gently stretches your back muscles and hamstrings.
- Can help relieve neck and jaw tension and headache.
- Encourages inward contemplation and self-awareness.

TIP

If you can't easily bring your torso to the bolster, add more blankets to bring the bolster to you so you can relax in the pose.

INSTRUCTIONS

1. Sit with your legs stretched out in front of you, with your feet about hip-width apart.
2. Place a block on its tallest setting between your shins. Set the narrow end of the bolster in your lap so that the other end rests on the block. Place the blanket on the bolster and lean forward, resting your abdomen, heart, and cheek on the bolster. Relax your arms by your sides.
3. Halfway through, turn your head and place the opposite cheek down for an equal stretch of your neck.
4. Remain in Supported Forward Fold for 5 to 8 minutes. To exit, press your hands into the bolster and sit up.

Supported Child's Pose

Forward Bend • 5 to 8 minutes

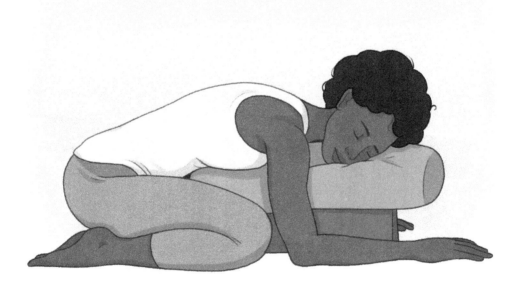

Bolster (or 2 rolled blankets or a large pillow)

2 blocks (or large hardcover books)

- If you are unable to bend your knees enough to support this pose, substitute Supported Forward Fold (page 36) or Supported Half Frog (page 80).

BENEFITS

- Supports and maintains your spine in normal, healthy flexion.
- Gently stretches your back muscles, glutes, and quadriceps muscles.
- Helps relieve back pain.
- Helps soothe anxiety and restlessness.
- Fosters a sense of calm and steadiness.

TIP

If your hips don't come all the way to your heels or you feel strain in your knees here, place folded blankets in the back of your knees for support.

INSTRUCTIONS

1. Come to your hands and knees and bring your big toes together. Keep your knees wide. Sit back on your heels and place one block between your knees and the other block just in front of it.
2. Place the bolster on the blocks so one end is between your knees.
3. Using your arms for support, bow forward onto the bolster and place your abdomen, heart, and either cheek on the bolster. Relax your arms.
4. Halfway through, turn your head and place the opposite cheek down for an equal stretch of your neck.
5. Remain in Supported Child's Pose for 5 to 8 minutes. To exit the pose, place your palms down on either side of the bolster and press down to lift up to sitting on your heels. Come onto your seat and stretch out your legs.

Reclining Butterfly

Hip Opener • 5 to 8 minutes

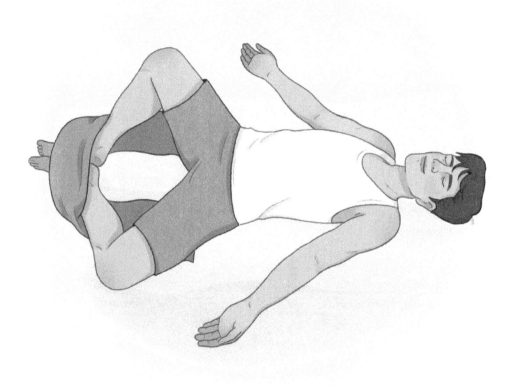

PROPS

Long eighth-fold blanket	Blanket roll

- If you are pregnant, substitute Pregnant Goddess Pose (page 86).
- If you experience discomfort in your knees or hips in this pose, use blocks or more blankets to prop up your thighs.

BENEFITS
- Supports and maintains your hips in gentle, healthy external rotation.
- Gently stretches your inner thigh muscles.
- Helps relieve hip pain due to long periods spent sitting.
- Encourages dual sensations of grounding and expansion.

INSTRUCTIONS

1. From a sitting position, place the long eighth-fold blanket behind you with the narrow end touching the base of your spine.
2. Bend your knees and bring the soles of your feet together, opening your knees wide to make a diamond shape with your legs.
3. Place the middle of the blanket roll on top of your feet, then draw the ends around your ankles to meet behind your heels so your outer shins are supported.
4. Using your hands for support, lie back onto the blanket behind you.
5. Remain in Reclining Butterfly for 5 to 8 minutes. To exit, use your hands to draw your knees together, then roll to one side and press yourself up to a sitting position.

Elevated Legs Up the Wall

Inversion • 5 to 10 minutes

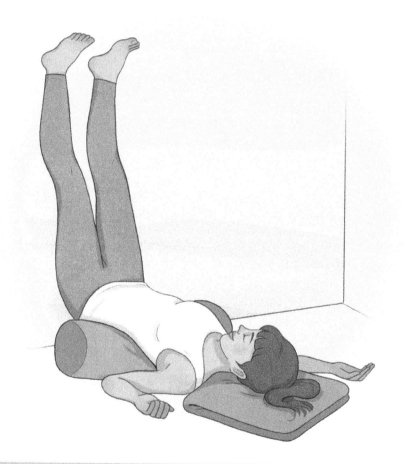

PROPS

Bolster (or 2 rolled blankets or a large pillow)

Square eighth-fold blanket

- Inverting is contraindicated for pregnancy, hernia, severe acid reflux, brain injuries, glaucoma, and high blood pressure. In these cases, substitute Legs Up the Bolster (page 82).
- If this pose aggravates your lower back, substitute Legs Up the Wall (page 62).

BENEFITS

- Supports your body in a gentle inversion, taking gravitational pressure off your legs and feet.
- Improves heart rate variability.
- Can alleviate swollen feet and tired legs.
- Soothes a frayed nervous system and tired mind.

TIP

If you've spent a long day on your feet, try this pose right before bed to relieve aches and pains in your legs and feet and calm your mind to prepare for a good night's sleep.

INSTRUCTIONS

1. Place the long edge of your bolster against the wall.
2. Sit on the bolster with one hip touching the wall; then, using your arms for support, lean back and gently swing your legs up the wall.
3. Lie back and use the blanket to support your head. Release your arms out wide.
4. Remain in Elevated Legs Up the Wall for 5 to 10 minutes. To exit, bend your knees into your chest and carefully roll off the bolster to one side, then press yourself up to a sitting position.

CHAPTER 4

Poses: Stress Relief

Mountain Brook

Backbend • 5 to 10 minutes

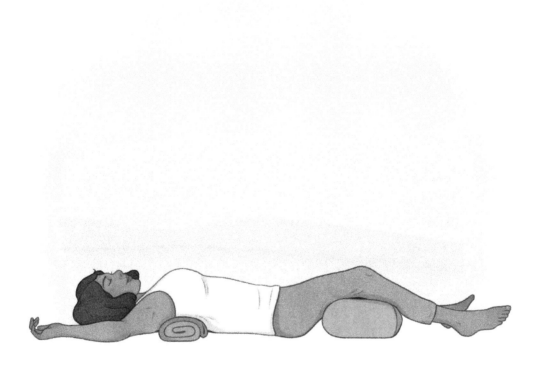

PRECAUTIONS

- Ensure that the blanket roll is placed behind your shoulder blades and spine to support the opening of your chest, and not in the lumbar curve of your lower back.

BENEFITS

- Supports and maintains your spine in normal, healthy extension.
- Gently stretches your chest and shoulders.
- Helps reverse the effects of long periods spent sitting and slouching.
- Invites your breath to deepen.
- Eases tension in your shoulders.
- Invites a sense of coolness and fluidity to temper the heat of stressful emotions.

TIP

Try to embody the name of this pose and imagine that your body is a river, flowing up and over each curve in the earth, feeling any resistance or tension wash downstream.

INSTRUCTIONS

1. From a sitting position, draw your legs over the bolster and place the blanket roll horizontally across the mat approximately one foot behind you.
2. Using your hands for support, relax your abdominals and lie back, adjusting the blanket roll so that it is behind your shoulder blades.
3. Take your arms out wide with your elbows bent in a cactus shape.
4. Remain in Mountain Brook for 5 to 10 minutes. To exit, bend your knees, place your feet on the bolster, and roll to one side. Press yourself up to a sitting position.

Supported Open Twist

Twist • 3 to 5 minutes per side

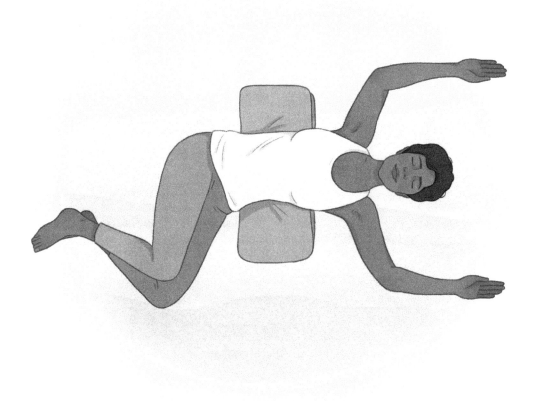

PROPS

Bolster (or 2 rolled blankets or a large pillow)

- If spinal rotation is contraindicated for you (in the case of spinal injury or pregnancy), skip this pose.
- If you experience lower back pain or sensitivity, substitute Gentle Open Twist (page 68).

BENEFITS

- Supports and maintains your spine in normal, healthy rotation.
- Gently decompresses your spine.
- Gently stretches the chest, shoulders, abdomen, and outer hip.
- Invites a sense of freedom and receptivity, transforming obstacles into possibility.

TIP

Breathing in twists can be challenging, as these poses place tension on the intercostal muscles between your ribs. Don't twist so far that you find that you cannot breathe easily, even if you feel that you can physically go further. Remember, you're here to relax.

INSTRUCTIONS

1. Start in Simple Supported Side Bend (page 28) with your right side on the bolster.
2. Leave your legs and hips as they are, and gently roll your left shoulder back into the twist.
3. Remain in Supported Open Twist for 3 to 5 minutes. To exit, gently return to Simple Supported Side Bend. Place your left hand onto the bolster in front of your heart and press yourself up.
4. Leave the bolster where it is and turn your body around to sitting on your left hip to repeat the pose on the second side.

Heart Pose with Butterfly Legs

Backbend, Hip Opener • 5 to 10 minutes

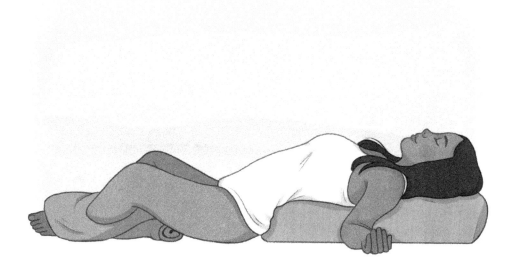

PROPS

Bolster (or 2 rolled blankets or a
large pillow)

Blanket roll

- If you suffer from lower back pain or sensitivity, substitute Pregnant Goddess Pose (page 86)

BENEFITS

- Supports and maintains natural, healthy spinal extension and external hip rotation.
- Gently stretches your chest, shoulders, and inner thigh muscles.
- Helps reverse the effects of sitting for long periods and slouching.
- Encourages a deep, calming breath.
- Helps alleviate the physical contraction of stress and anger.
- Instills renewed energy and mental clarity.

TIP

If you feel your heart racing in response to the stretch across your chest, make your exhales longer than your inhales and feel your heart slow down again as you relax.

INSTRUCTIONS

1. From a sitting position, bring the narrow end of the bolster up to the base of your spine.
2. Bend your knees and bring the soles of your feet together, opening your knees wide to make a diamond shape with your legs.
3. Place the middle of the blanket roll on top of your feet, then draw the ends around your ankles to meet behind your heels so your outer shins are supported.
4. Reach behind you and hold the bolster with both hands. Relax your abdominal muscles and gently lower your spine and back of your head down onto the bolster. Release your arms wide.
5. Remain in the pose for 5 to 10 minutes. To exit, use your hands to draw your knees together. Place one hand down on the earth next to you and gently roll to one side, then press yourself up to a sitting position.

Extended Supported Bridge

Backbend, Inversion • 8 to 10 minutes

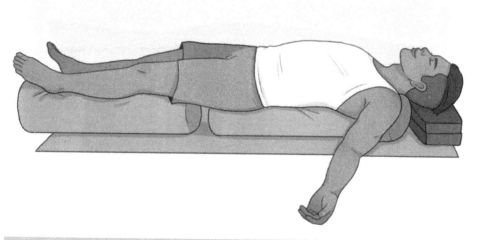

2 bolsters (or make 2 from 4 rolled blankets or 2 large pillows)

Block (or large hardcover book or a pillow)

- Inverting is contraindicated for pregnancy, hernia, severe acid reflux, brain injuries, glaucoma, and high blood pressure. In these cases, substitute Legs Up the Bolster (page 82).
- Ensure the bolsters are wide enough for you to feel stable and supported.
- If you're tall, you may need additional support for your feet.

BENEFITS

- Gently stretches your neck, chest, and shoulders.
- Eases tension in your neck and jaw.
- Invites a sense of weightlessness.

TIP

Stay present to the abundance of support that is available to your heart and feel your body melt into the bolsters as stress and tension roll off your shoulders.

INSTRUCTIONS

1. Place two bolsters end to end with the block at one end for your head.
2. Carefully sit on the bolster closest to the block and extend your legs along the other bolster.
3. Using your hands for support, lie back so that your head is resting on the block, and the rest of your body is supported by the bolsters. Release your arms.
4. Remain in Extended Supported Bridge for 8 to 10 minutes. To exit, bend your knees, place one hand down on the ground next to you, and gently roll off the bolsters.

Supported Straddle Forward Fold

Forward Bend • 5 to 8 minutes

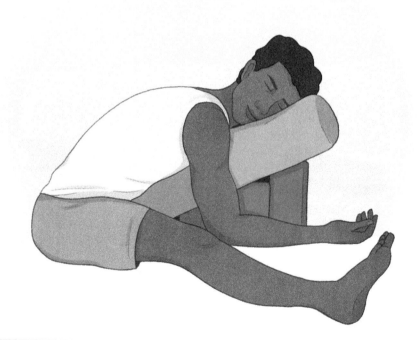

PROPS

Bolster (or 2 rolled blankets or a large pillow)

2 blocks (or large hardcover books)

- If you have any injury or strain to your hamstring tendons, substitute Seated Butterfly (page 74).
- You may need to stack a second bolster or folded blankets on top of the bolster so you can avoid strain and relax.

- Gently stretches your glutes, hamstrings, and inner thigh and back muscles.
- Eases tension in your neck and jaw.
- Relieves tension in your lower back.
- Grounds your energy and centers your mind.

TIP

Bring your awareness down to the roots of your body, and feel your hips, legs, and feet softening as the stirrings of your mind subside.

INSTRUCTIONS

1. Start in a sitting position with your legs long and wide.
2. Place a block about one foot from your pelvis on its lowest setting. On the far side of it, place another block on its tallest setting, creating an "L" shape.
3. Secure the bolster on top of the blocks with one end close to your pelvis, then lean forward and rest your abdomen, chest, and either cheek on the bolster. Relax your arms.
4. Halfway through, turn your head and place the opposite cheek down for an equal stretch of your neck.
5. Remain in Supported Straddle Forward Fold for 5 to 8 minutes. To exit, press yourself up, move the props aside, and use your hands to bend your knees into your chest.

Reclining Pigeon

Hip Opener • 3 to 5 minutes per side

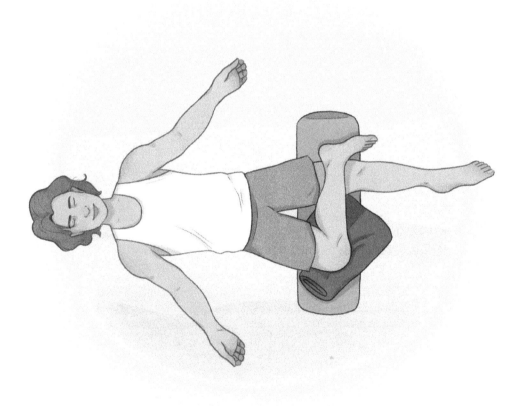

PROPS

Bolster (or 2 rolled blankets or a large pillow)

Square eighth-fold blanket, folded in half

- Gently stretches your inner thigh muscles.
- Supports your hip in a healthy, normal external rotation.
- Relieves tension associated with long periods of sitting or standing.
- Invites a sense of deep peace as the muscles that are stimulated by fight-or-flight relax and open.

Studies have revealed a mysterious connection between tension in your hips and your jaw, perhaps because both areas contain muscles associated with the fight-or-flight response. Relax your jaw and feel tension melt away from your hips in this pose.

INSTRUCTIONS

1. From a sitting position, bring both legs over the bolster. Place a folded blanket next to your right knee.
2. Cross your right ankle just above your left knee so your legs make a "figure 4" shape, then tuck the blanket under your right thigh for support.
3. Using your hands for support, lie back and release your arms by your sides.
4. Remain in Reclining Pigeon for 3 to 5 minutes. To exit, use your right hand to draw your right knee up, then bring both knees in toward your chest and roll to one side. Press yourself up to a sitting position and change sides to repeat the pose.

Reclining Butterfly with Feet on the Bolster

Hip Opener • 5 to 8 minutes

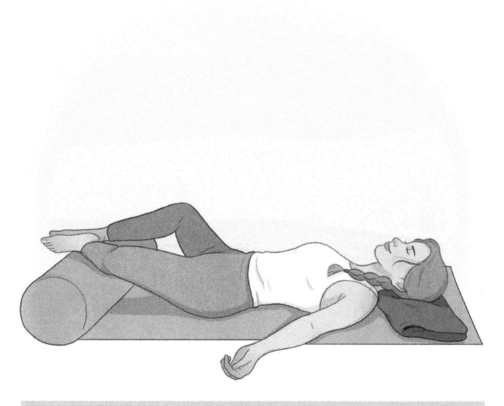

PROPS

Bolster (or 2 rolled blankets or a large pillow)

Square eighth-fold blanket

- If this pose aggravates your hips, substitute Reclining Butterfly (page 40).

BENEFITS
- Supports and maintains your hips in a gentle, healthy external rotation.
- Gently stretches your inner thigh muscles.
- Helps relieve hip pain due to long periods spent sitting, standing, or walking.
- Can alleviate lower back tension associated with tightness in your hips and pelvis.
- Encourages mental tranquility and rejuvenates your mind.

TIP

Stress can make you feel defensive or closed off. Focus on the natural, easy sense of opening your body is experiencing and let your mind and energy absorb that same energy.

INSTRUCTIONS

1. Position the bolster lengthwise near your feet. Lie back and bring your feet up onto the bolster. Place the soles of your feet together and let your knees open wide so that your outer shins rest on the bolster.
2. You can reduce the intensity of the stretch by moving your hips farther away from the bolster, so your knees aren't bent at as deep of an angle.
3. Support your head and neck on the blanket and relax your arms at your sides.
4. Remain here for 5 to 8 minutes. To exit, use your hands to draw your knees together, roll to one side, then press yourself up to a sitting position.

Restorative Frog

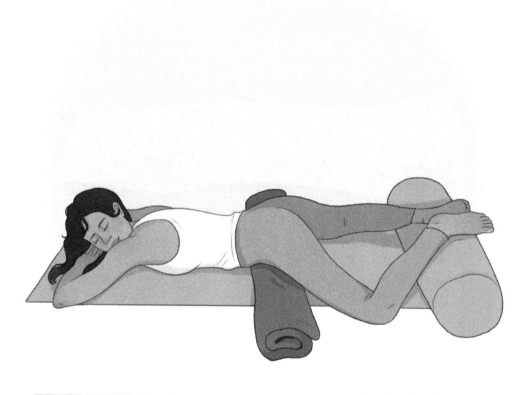

PROPS

Bolster (or 2 rolled blankets or a large pillow)

Blanket roll

- If the blanket roll creates any pressure in your lower back, remove it.
- If you are in your second or third trimester of pregnancy, substitute Pregnant Goddess Pose (page 86).
- If you lack the hip mobility for this pose, substitute Supported Half Frog (page 80).

BENEFITS

- Gently stretches your groin muscles and inner thighs to relieve tension.
- Helps prevent groin strain if you are tight in this area.
- Lying facedown has been found to improve oxygenation and respiration.
- Invites a blissful sense of support, connection, and nurturing.

TIP

Try placing your forehead on your hands here and close your eyes, bringing your awareness to the center of your forehead. Feel your inner gaze opening and let critical thinking give way to your natural intuition.

INSTRUCTIONS

1. Start on hands and knees with the bolster just behind your feet, and the blanket roll laid horizontally across your mat between your hands and knees.
2. Carefully lower yourself down onto your abdomen so that the blanket roll supports your pelvis.
3. Bend your knees and bring your feet together and knees wide, placing the inner edges of your feet on the bolster. Feel free to move the bolster farther away or closer to you until you feel supported.
4. Make a pillow with your hands and rest one cheek down. Halfway through, turn your head and place the opposite cheek down for an equal stretch in your neck.
5. Remain in Restorative Frog for 3 to 5 minutes. To exit, kick the bolster out of your way using your feet and extend your legs out long behind you. Press up to hands and knees and come to a seated position.

Legs Up the Wall

Inversion • 5 to 10 minutes

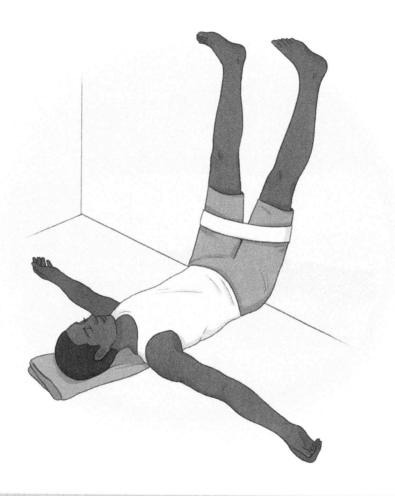

Yoga strap | Square eighth-fold blanket

- If you are pregnant or find this pose irritates your hamstrings, substitute Legs Up the Bolster (page 82).

BENEFITS

- Supports your body in a gentle inversion, taking gravitational pressure off your legs and feet.
- Gently stretches your hamstrings.
- Helps alleviate swollen feet and tired legs.
- Soothes a frayed nervous system and tired mind.
- Can improve sleep, which in turn can reduce feelings of fatigue.

TIP

This is a great pose you can do while on a layover. At the airport, find a quiet corner and enjoy a few minutes with your feet up and feel the stress of travel melt away.

INSTRUCTIONS

1. Secure the yoga strap around your thighs so there's a small gap between your legs.
2. Sit with one hip touching the wall, then, using your hands for support, lean back and gently swing your legs up the wall. Let them relax into the support of the yoga strap instead of trying to keep them together.
3. Support your head and neck with the blanket and relax your arms at your sides.
4. Remain in Legs Up the Wall for 5 to 10 minutes. To exit, bend your knees into your chest and roll onto one side. Press yourself up to a sitting position and remove the yoga strap.

CHAPTER 5

Poses: Pain Relief

Supported Heart Pose with Legs Over a Bolster

Backbend • 8 to 12 minutes

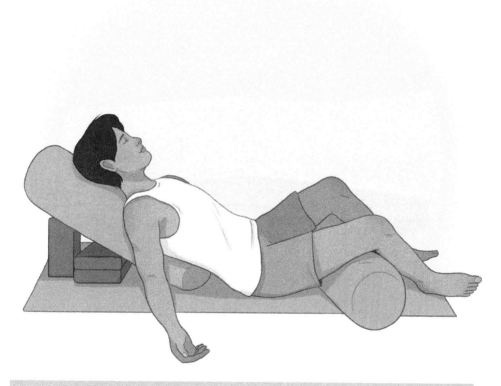

PROPS

2 bolsters (or make 2 from 4 rolled blankets or 2 large pillows)

2 blocks (or large hardcover books)

- Gently opens your chest and shoulders without irritating your lower back.
- Softens your psoas, the deep hip flexor muscles that can become chronically contracted if you spend extended periods sitting.
- Relieves lower back pain associated with tight hip flexors.
- Allows anyone with back pain or injury to experience a supported heart opener.
- Brings about feelings of safety and comfort within your body.

TIP

There's nothing restorative about taking a tumble. When it comes to setting up this pose, always take a moment to ensure the bolster and the blocks are stable. The blocks are steadier than you think, but hold the bolster behind you with both hands before lying back so you feel secure. If you still feel unsteady, you can always prop your bolster up on top of one or two large pillows instead of blocks. The most important thing is that you feel safe, supported, and relaxed.

INSTRUCTIONS

1. Set up your bolster on 2 blocks, one higher than the other so your bolster is on a diagonal, with one edge securely on the ground.
2. About a foot or so away, position the second bolster perpendicular to the angled bolster. Sit with the base of your spine touching the end of the angled bolster and draw your legs over the other bolster.
3. Hold the bolster behind you with both hands, relax your abdominals, and gently release yourself back. Relax your arms to the side.
4. Remain here for 8 to 12 minutes. To exit, place your palms down next to your hips, lift your head, and then gently press your lower back into the bolster to come up to a sitting position.

Gentle Open Twist

Twist • 3 to 5 minutes per side

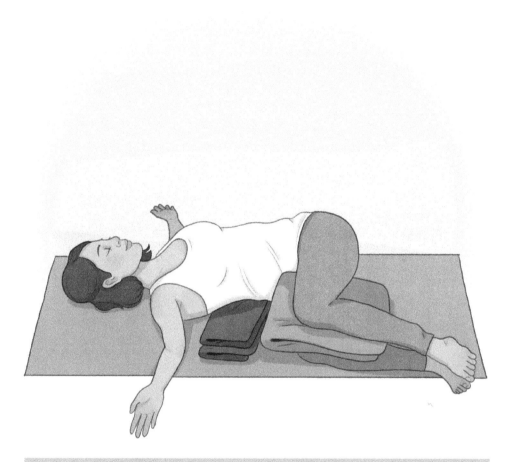

2 long eighth-fold blankets | Square eighth-fold blanket

- If spinal rotation is contraindicated for you, in the case of spinal injury or pregnancy, skip this pose.

BENEFITS

- Supports and maintains your spine in healthy, normal rotation.
- Gently stretches your chest, shoulders, and outer hip.
- Gently decompresses your spine.
- Helps relieve lower back and hip pain associated with tight spinal extensors, excessive periods of sitting, standing, or walking.

TIP

Although it's most likely just an energetic association and not a physical benefit, many people find that twists feel replenishing. Imagine each exhale releasing tightness and pain, and each inhale inviting in healing and rejuvenation.

INSTRUCTIONS

1. Stack the 2 long eighth-fold blankets across the top third of your mat.
2. Sit with your right hip touching the bottom long edge of the blankets with your knees bent and feet tucked in behind you.
3. Place the square eighth-fold blanket between your knees for comfort.
4. Slide your right hand away from your right hip to bring your right side onto the stacked blankets, coming into a Simple Supported Side Bend (page 28). Use your right arm as a pillow.
5. When you're ready, keep your hips and legs as they are and gently roll your left shoulder back turning your chest toward the sky. Take your arms out wide to support the spacious feeling in your chest.
6. Remain in Gentle Open Twist for 3 to 5 minutes. To exit, return to Simple Supported Side Bend, then press your left hand down to come up to a sitting position. Leave your props as they are and turn your body around to sitting on your left hip to repeat the pose on the other side.

Restorative Tree

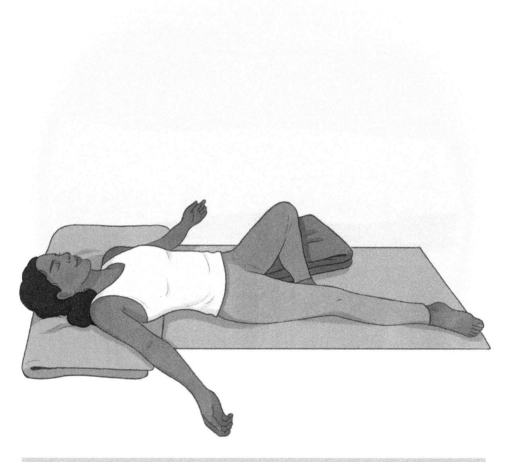

PROPS

Quarter-fold blanket	Square eighth-fold blanket

- Gently stretches your groin and inner thigh muscles.
- Supports your hip in healthy, normal external rotation.
- Helps relieve lower back and hip pain associated with tight psoas, the deep hip flexor muscles that can become chronically contracted if you spend extended periods sitting.

INSTRUCTIONS

1. Lie back and support your head and neck with the quarter-fold blanket.
2. Place the square eighth-fold blanket next to your right hip, then bend your right knee and bring the sole of your foot to your inner left thigh. Lower your knee to the side and adjust the blanket so it supports your outer thigh. If there's still space between your thigh and the blanket, roll it up so it properly supports your leg.
3. Relax your arms out to the side.
4. Remain in Restorative Tree Pose for 5 minutes. To exit, use your right hand to draw your knee back to center. Move the blanket to the left side and use it to support your left leg to repeat the pose on the other side.

Seated Half Butterfly

Hip Opener, Forward Fold • 5 minutes per side

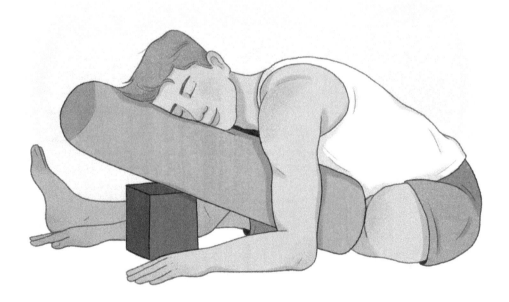

Bolster (or 2 rolled blankets or a large pillow)

Block (or large hardcover book)

- If you should avoid forward bending due to injury or pain, substitute Head to Bolster Pose (page 76).
- If you experience pain or discomfort in your lower back in forward bends, use more support such as two bolsters, or rest your head and arms on a chair seat to minimize spinal flexion.

BENEFITS

- Gently stretches your back, glutes, groin, and inner thigh muscles.
- Helps relieve lower back pain associated with tight spinal extensors and lordosis.
- Can help alleviate neck pain, headache, and menstrual pain.

TIP

If you need a quick stress relief break at the office, you can use the seat of any chair without wheels to support your arms and head in this pose.

INSTRUCTIONS

1. From a sitting position, bend your right knee and draw your heel toward your pelvis. Extend your left leg long and wide.
2. Place the block in front of you and rest the bolster on it, keeping the narrow end close to your right foot.
3. Bow forward and rest your chest and one cheek on the bolster.
4. Remain in Seated Half Butterfly for 5 minutes. To exit, press into your hands and sit up. Move the bolster out of your way so you can extend your right leg and bend your left knee to repeat the pose on the other side.

Seated Butterfly

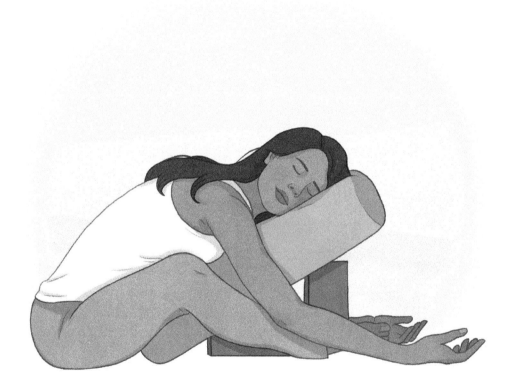

PROPS

Bolster (or 2 rolled blankets or a large pillow)

2 blocks (or large hardcover books)

- If you should avoid forward bending due to injury or pain, substitute Head to Bolster Pose (page 76).
- If you experience pain or discomfort in your lower back in forward bends, use more support such as two bolsters, or rest your head and arms on a chair seat to minimize spinal flexion.

BENEFITS

- Supports and maintains your spine in healthy, normal flexion.
- Gently stretches your back, glutes, groin, and inner thigh muscles.
- Helps relieve lower back pain associated with tight spinal extensors, lordosis, and pregnancy.
- Can help alleviate neck pain, headache, and menstrual pain.

TIP

If you experience pain or discomfort in your hips or knees here, place pillows or blankets underneath your outer thighs for support.

INSTRUCTIONS

1. From a seated position, bring the soles of your feet together and let your knees fall apart wide. Then move your feet apart so you can place a block between them on its tallest setting.
2. Place the second block on its lowest setting closer to your pelvis.
3. Rest the bolster onto the blocks and bow forward to rest your chest and one cheek on the bolster.
4. Halfway through, turn your head and place the opposite cheek down for an equal stretch of your neck.
5. Remain in Seated Butterfly for 5 to 8 minutes. To exit the pose, press into your hands to sit up and move the blocks aside to stretch out your legs.

Head to Bolster Pose

Hip Opener, Forward Fold • 5 to 8 minutes

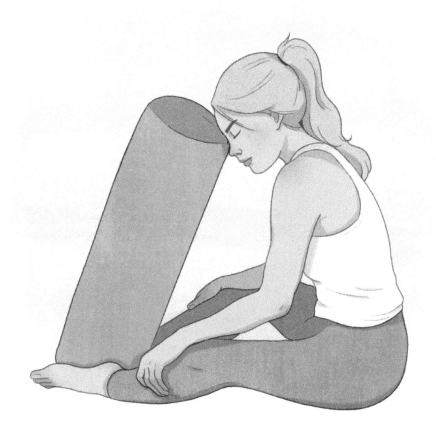

Bolster (or 2 rolled blankets or a large pillow)

- Gently stretches your back, glutes, groin, and inner thigh muscles.
- Allows those with spinal injury and those in the late stages of pregnancy to enjoy gentle forward folding.
- Can help alleviate neck pain, headache, and jaw pain.

Bring your awareness to the center of your forehead and allow the gentle pressure of the bolster to ease tension in your temples and jaw.

INSTRUCTIONS

1. From a sitting position, bring the soles of your feet together and let your knees fall apart wide. Then move your feet apart so you can place the end of the bolster between them.
2. Draw the other end of the bolster toward you and rest your forehead on it. Relax your arms.
3. Remain in Head to Bolster Pose for 5 to 8 minutes. To exit, hold the bolster with your hands and lift your head.

Supported Pigeon

Hip Opener • 3 to 5 minutes per side

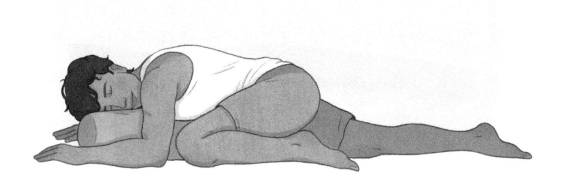

PROPS

Bolster (or 2 rolled blankets or a large pillow)

- If you have a knee injury, substitute Reclining Pigeon (page 56).

BENEFITS

- Gently stretches your hip rotators including the piriformis muscle, and hip flexors such as the psoas muscle, the deep hip flexor muscles that can become chronically contracted if you spend extended periods sitting.
- Supports your hips in healthy, normal external rotation, countering the effects of sitting and walking.
- Can alleviate lower back, hip, and sciatic nerve pain.

TIP

Irritation of the sciatic nerve (which travels from your lower back down the back of each leg) can produce a burning sensation from your buttocks down your legs. This irritation can be caused by a disc injury (in which case you should see a doctor) or a tight piriformis muscle, which is a small muscle deep in your buttocks. Fortunately, the latter can be relieved by gentle and regular stretching of the piriformis, through poses like Supported Pigeon. If you suffer from sciatic pain and find this pose offers relief, do it daily.

INSTRUCTIONS

1. Come to your hands and knees with the bolster out long in front of you. Slide your right knee forward, keeping the bolster inside your knee, and your left knee back.
2. Adjust the bolster so it touches your pelvis, then bow forward so it supports the front of your left hip, your torso, and either cheek.
3. Remain in Supported Pigeon for 3 to 5 minutes. To exit, press your hands down and slide your right knee back to come back to hands and knees. Change sides and repeat the pose on the other side.

Supported Half Frog

Hip Opener • 3 to 5 minutes per side

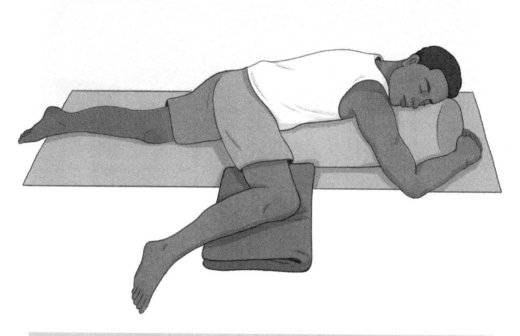

Bolster (or 2 rolled blankets or a large pillow)

Long eighth-fold blanket

- Gently stretches your groin and inner thigh muscles.
- Helps relieve lower back pain and menstrual pain.

If you experience pain or discomfort in your inner thigh or hip, draw your knee up higher toward your armpit.

INSTRUCTIONS

1. Come to your hands and knees with the bolster vertically in front of you. Place the blanket to the right of the bolster.
2. Lower your hips and torso onto the bolster.
3. Keep your left leg extended behind you and bend your right knee to the side so you can rest it on the blanket.
4. Your knee should be bent to roughly 90 degrees and in line with your hip.
5. Place one cheek on the bolster and gently wrap your arms around the far end of the bolster.
6. Remain in Supported Half Frog for 3 to 5 minutes. To exit, press your hands down, slide your right knee back, and return to hands and knees. Change sides to repeat the pose on the other side.

Legs Up the Bolster

Inversion • 5 to 10 minutes

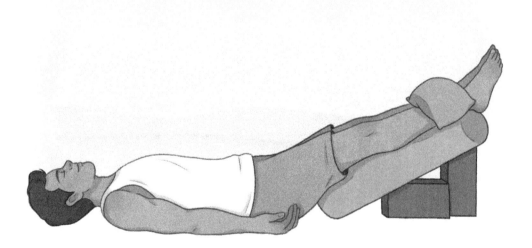

PROPS

Bolster (or 2 rolled
blankets or
a large pillow)

2 blocks (or large
hardcover books)

Yoga sandbag (or a
heavy folded blanket)

- If you suffer from severe congestive heart failure or peripheral arterial disease, skip this pose.

BENEFITS
- Supports your body in a gentle inversion, taking gravitational pressure off your legs and feet without straining your hamstrings.
- Can alleviate pain in your legs and feet associated with swelling, pregnancy, and long periods of standing.

TIP

Your hips should be close enough to the bolster that the backs of your legs are completely supported and there is no space behind your knees or thighs to ensure that you don't hyperextend your knees.

INSTRUCTIONS

1. Set up 2 blocks with one on the tallest setting and the other on the lowest setting. Place the bolster onto the blocks so that it is on a diagonal with one end touching the floor.
2. From a sitting position, bring one hip up to the edge of the bolster, then, using your hands for support, lean back a little and draw your legs up onto the bolster. Place the sandbag on top of your ankles so your legs can relax without rolling off the bolster.
3. Lie back and relax your arms to the side.
4. Remain in Legs Up the Bolster for 5 to 10 minutes. To exit, remove the sandbag, bend one knee and then the other, place your feet on the bolster, then roll to your side and press yourself up to a sitting position.

CHAPTER 6

Poses: Other Poses for Healing

Pregnant Goddess Pose

Opening Pose, Backbend, Hip Opener • 8 to 12 minutes

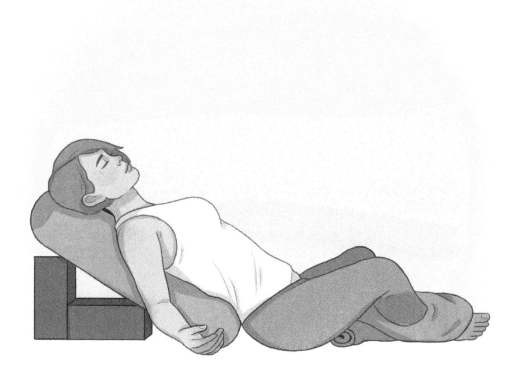

PROPS

Bolster (or 2 rolled blankets or a large pillow)

Blanket roll

2 blocks (or large hardcover books)

PRECAUTIONS

- If you experience discomfort in your knees or hips in this pose, extend your legs out long.

BENEFITS

- Provides a safe, gentle, and much-needed opening of your chest, shoulders, and inner thigh muscles during pregnancy.
- Allows you to feel comfortable and supported without overstretching during pregnancy.
- Improves respiration.
- Helps relieve stress and anxiety during pregnancy—and beyond.
- Provides a safe and supportive alternative to Basic Relaxation Pose (page 26) and other backbends during pregnancy.

INSTRUCTIONS

1. Set up your bolster on 2 blocks, one higher than the other so that your bolster is on a diagonal, with one edge securely on the ground.
2. Sit with the base of your spine touching the end of the bolster on the ground. Bend your knees and bring the soles of your feet together, opening your knees wide to make a diamond shape with your legs.
3. Place the middle of the blanket roll on top of your feet, then draw the ends around your ankles to meet behind your heels so your outer shins are supported.
4. Reach behind you and hold the bolster with both hands, so you can be sure it is steady before you lie back onto the bolster behind you.
5. Remain in Pregnant Goddess for 8 to 12 minutes, longer if you are comfortable. To exit, use your hands to draw your knees together then roll to your left side and press yourself up to a sitting position.

Side Lying Pose

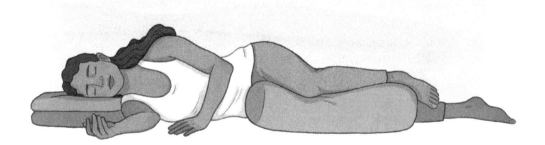

PROPS

2 square eighth-fold blankets	Bolster (or 2 rolled blankets or a large pillow)

- If you are pregnant, only take Side Lying Pose on your left side during pregnancy to avoid compression of the inferior vena cava.
- If you suffer from sciatic or low back pain and Side Lying Pose on one side increases your discomfort, only practice this pose on the other side.

BENEFITS

- Offers a safe and comfortable alternative to Basic Relaxation Pose (page 26) if you are pregnant, or if lying on your back causes you discomfort.
- Provides a cozy alternative to Basic Relaxation Pose (page 26) or any of the supported backbends in this book if you feel too vulnerable lying on your back.
- Helps relieve pain and discomfort in your lower back.

INSTRUCTIONS

1. Stack the 2 blankets to create ample support for your head.
2. Lie down on your left side using the blankets as a pillow. Let your left arm extend out onto the ground in front of you.
3. Keep your left leg mostly straight, and bend your right knee resting your inner thigh and shin on the bolster. Relax.
4. Remain in Side Lying Pose for 5 to 8 minutes. To exit, press into your right hand to come up and turn over to lie down and repeat the pose on your right side (unless you are pregnant).

Supported Bridge

Backbend, Inversion • 3 to 5 minutes

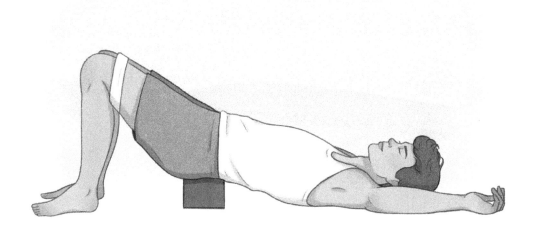

PROPS

Yoga strap

Block (or a large hardcover book)

- If you experience pain or discomfort in your lower back during this pose, substitute Extended Supported Bridge Pose (page 52) or Single Leg Up the Chair (page 98) for a gentle hip flexor stretch.

BENEFITS

- Supports your spine in very gentle extension.
- Provides a welcome stretch across your hip flexors and belly during pregnancy.
- Relieves the effects of extended periods spent sitting.
- Improves respiration.
- The gentle pressure of the block against your sacrum can help alleviate lower back pain.

TIP

Make sure the block is placed under your sacrum, at the base of your spine, and not in the lumbar curve of your lower back.

INSTRUCTIONS

1. Secure the yoga strap around your thighs so there's a small gap between your legs and they are not touching.
2. Lie on your back with your knees bent and your feet on the ground. Press into your feet and lift your hips up, placing the block on its lowest setting underneath your sacrum.
3. Let your legs relax into the support of the yoga strap. Take your arms out into a cactus position and relax.
4. Remain in Supported Bridge for 3 to 5 minutes. To exit, press your feet down and lift your hips enough to remove the block. Lower your hips and hug your knees to your chest. Remove the yoga strap from your legs and roll to one side, then press yourself up to a sitting position.

Reclining Hero Pose

Backbend • 3 to 5 minutes

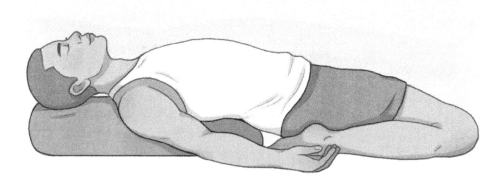

PROPS

Bolster (or 2 rolled blankets or a large pillow)

- Reclining Hero Pose may not be suitable for all bodies; do this pose only if you can easily sit with your hips on the ground between your feet.
- If you experience pain or discomfort in your knees or lower back in this pose, substitute with Supported Bridge (page 90).
- If you are pregnant, do this pose with your bolster stacked on two blocks as shown in Pregnant Goddess Pose (page 86) to reduce the curve in your lower back.

BENEFITS

- Supports your spine in extension.
- Provides a delicious stretch across your knees, quadriceps, hip flexors, belly, and chest.
- Relieves the effects of extended periods spent sitting.
- Improves respiration.

> **TIP**
>
> If this pose is accessible but does not feel restorative to you, try using two bolsters, or stacking folded blankets on your bolster for additional support.

INSTRUCTIONS

1. Start on your hands and knees with the bolster laid out the long way behind your toes. Bring your knees together and your feet wide enough to sit in between them.
2. Using your hands for support, lie back onto the bolster behind you. Relax your arms to the sides.
3. Remain in Reclining Hero for 3 to 5 minutes. To exit, lift your head, then use your arms to press yourself up. Come to a sitting position and stretch your legs out in front of you.

Heart Pose with a Chair

Backbend • 3 to 5 minutes

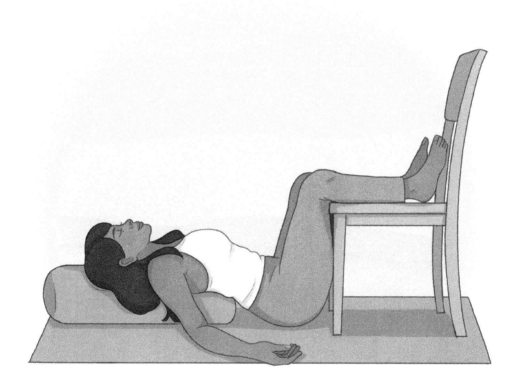

PROPS

Bolster (or 2 rolled blankets or a large pillow)

Chair

- If you feel pain or discomfort in your lower back in this pose, substitute Legs Up the Chair (page 100).

BENEFITS

- Supports your spine in extension.
- Softens your psoas muscles, the deep hip flexor muscles that can become chronically contracted if you spend extended periods sitting, and gently opens your chest and shoulders to relieve the effects of extended periods spent sitting.
- Improves respiration.
- Provides an accessible, lower back–friendly alternative to Heart Pose (page 34).

TIP

If you can bring a bolster to the office, this pose makes a great afternoon pick-me-up during a long day spent sitting in front of a computer.

INSTRUCTIONS

1. Start in a sitting position with the bolster touching the base of your spine and the chair in front of you.
2. Reach behind you and hold the bolster to stabilize it, then lie back.
3. Bring your calves up onto the chair seat one at a time. Release your arms by your sides.
4. Remain here for 3 to 5 minutes. To exit, bring both legs carefully down to one side, and use your hands to support you as you roll off the bolster onto your side. Press yourself up to a sitting position.

Chair Forward Fold

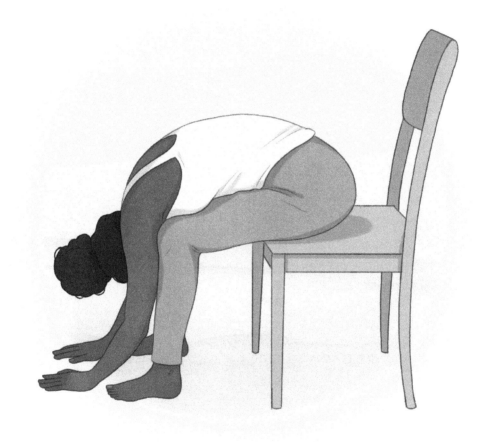

PROPS

Chair

- If you should avoid all spinal forward bends, skip this pose and substitute Legs Up the Chair (page 100).
- Inverting is contraindicated for pregnancy, hernia, severe acid reflux, brain injuries, glaucoma, and high blood pressure.

BENEFITS
- Supports your spine in flexion.
- Stretches your glutes and back muscles.
- Helps relieve tension in your neck, shoulders, and jaw.
- This is a forward fold you can do anywhere, from the conference room at work to the airport during a long travel day.

TIP

If tightness in your back doesn't allow your torso to come all the way to your thighs, place folded blankets in your lap for support.

INSTRUCTIONS

1. Start sitting on the chair with your feet flat on the ground, about six inches apart.
2. Draw your chin to your chest, let your shoulders round forward, and slowly roll down until your torso is resting on your thighs and your head is hanging between your knees. Widen your legs if needed.
3. Release your hands onto the ground. Relax your neck and jaw.
4. Remain in Chair Forward Fold for up to 3 minutes. To exit, bring your hands onto your knees and press down to roll up to a sitting position.

Single Leg Up the Chair

Hip Opener • 5 to 7 minutes per side

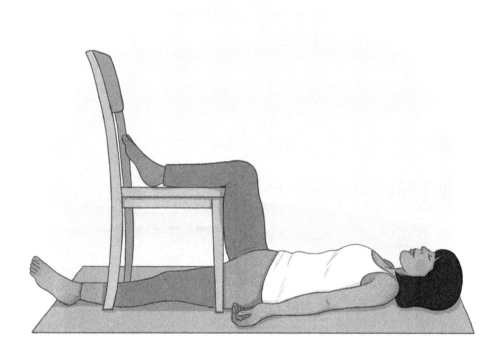

Chair

- Releases your hip flexor and groin muscles.
- Helps relieve lower back, hip, and knee pain.
- Supports your pelvis in a neutral alignment.

Hip flexor muscles like the psoas are sometimes contracted because they're compensating for patterns of instability in your core, spine, or breath, and deep stretching doesn't always help. In this pose, focus on simply releasing your hip flexors and abdomen and notice how your breath opens up in response.

INSTRUCTIONS

1. Start in a sitting position with your knees bent, close to the chair. Extend your right leg out long, in between the legs of the chair.
2. Place your hands behind you and lean back enough to gently swing your left leg up onto the chair seat.
3. Carefully lie back with your right leg extended on the ground between the chair legs, and the left calf resting on the chair seat. Release your arms by your sides.
4. Remain here for 5 to 7 minutes. To exit the pose, use your left foot to gently slide the chair out of your way, roll to one side, and press yourself up to a sitting position, then repeat the pose on the other side.

Legs Up the Chair

Inversions • 5 to 10 minutes

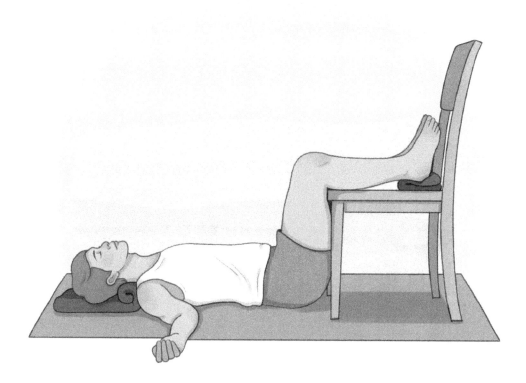

PROPS

Chair

Square eighth-fold blanket

PRECAUTIONS

• Inverting is contraindicated for pregnancy, hernia, severe acid reflux, brain injuries, glaucoma, and high blood pressure.

BENEFITS

• Supports your body in a gentle, simple inversion without irritating your hamstrings.
• Softens your hip flexor muscles.
• Can alleviate swollen feet and tired legs.

INSTRUCTIONS

1. Start in a sitting position with one hip close to the chair.
2. Using your hands for support, lean back and draw both calves up onto the chair seat, then ease yourself down onto your back.
3. Support your head with the blanket and release your arms by your sides.
4. Remain in Legs Up the Chair for 5 to 10 minutes. To exit, draw your knees in and roll to one side. Press yourself up to a sitting position.

Seated Meditation Pose

Hip Opener, Finishing Pose • 3 to 5 minutes

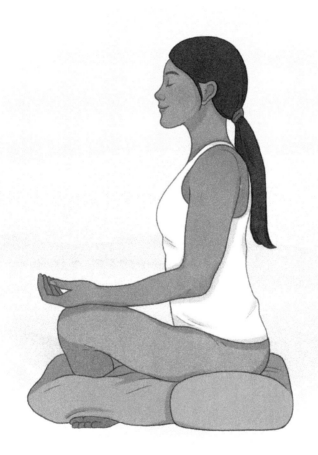

Bolster (or 2 rolled blankets or a large pillow)

Blanket roll

BENEFITS

- Supports your hips in gentle external rotation.
- Empowers you to sit confidently and comfortably
  for meditation.
- Brings gentle awareness to your spine.

TIP

Seated meditation can be intimidating, and sitting cross-legged can be more challenging than it appears. I recommend saving this pose for the end of your practice, so both your body and mind are well prepared for the physicality of sitting and the mental quietude of meditation.

INSTRUCTIONS

1. Sit on the bolster.
2. Bend your knees and cross your legs.
3. Place the blanket roll in front of your shins, then tuck the ends under your outer thighs for support so your knees are level with your hips.
4. Rest your hands on your knees and close your eyes. Use one of the breathing exercises or meditations described in Chapter 8 (page 147), or simply bring your awareness to your breath.
5. Remain in Seated Meditation Pose for 3 to 5 minutes, longer if you are still comfortable. To exit, use your hands to draw your knees together, then stretch your legs out long.

CHAPTER 7

Sequences

This chapter contains restorative yoga sequences designed for you to follow, each with a different therapeutic focus, as well as tips for building your own sequence. Although some of the sequences are suggested for a specific time of day, you can do any of these sequences whenever it works for your schedule. You may choose a sequence based on your physical needs, emotional state, or how much time you have available.

In the beginning of your journey, try out as many of the sequences as you can and when you find ones that work for you, bookmark them so you can incorporate them into your regular routine.

Remember that in addition to the listed props, for each sequence you'll need your yoga mat, blankets to cover your mat and yourself, and an eye pillow (or washcloth) to cover your eyes.

From Effort to Ease

The basic restorative yoga sequence • 55 to 85 minutes

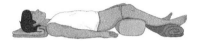

Basic Relaxation Pose

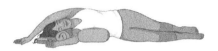

Simple Supported Side Bend

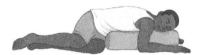

Grounding Spinal Twist

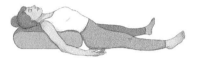

Heart Pose

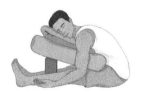

Supported Forward Fold

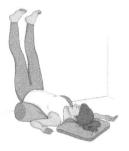

Elevated Legs Up the Wall

PROPS	POSES
• Bolster (or two rolled blankets or a large pillow) • Blanket roll • Block (or large hardcover book) • Square eighth-fold blanket	• Basic Relaxation Pose (page 26) • Simple Supported Side Bend (page 28) • Grounding Spinal Twist (page 30) • Heart Pose (page 34) • Supported Forward Fold (page 36) • Elevated Legs Up the Wall (page 42)

- If you experience lower back pain or discomfort in Heart Pose, substitute Supported Heart Pose with Legs Over a Bolster (page 66).
- If you are pregnant or suffer from hernia, severe acid reflux, brain injuries, glaucoma, or high blood pressure, skip Elevated Legs Up the Wall.

TIP

In Basic Relaxation Pose, use the Body Scan meditation outlined in Chapter 8 (page 147) to help relax your entire body.

BENEFITS

- Gently moves your spine to reduce pain and enhance mobility.
- Releases tension and recharges your body and mind.

INSTRUCTIONS

1. Set up your mat so the narrow end is close to the wall.
2. Begin with 20 to 30 minutes in **Basic Relaxation Pose**, then bend your knees and roll to your side.
3. Press yourself up to a sitting position, then move your legs off the bolster to the left so you are sitting on your right hip with your right thigh running along the edge of the bolster and your feet tucked in behind you. Guide yourself into **Simple Supported Side Bend** for 3 to 5 minutes.
4. Leave your props as they are and turn yourself around to repeat the pose on the other side. After you've completed both sides, press yourself up and turn the bolster so it's lengthwise with the narrow end touching your left hip. Guide yourself into **Grounding Spinal Twist** for 3 to 5 minutes.
5. Leave your props as they are and turn yourself around to repeat the pose on the other side. After you've completed both sides, press yourself up, leave your bolster where it is, and come to a sitting position with the base of your spine touching the narrow end of the bolster and your legs extended. Guide yourself into **Heart Pose** for 5 to 10 minutes.
6. Bend your knees, roll to one side and press yourself up to a sitting position. Turn back around to face your bolster, position your block and blanket, and move into **Supported Forward Fold** for 5 to 8 minutes.
7. To complete the practice, move your bolster to the wall for **Elevated Legs Up the Wall** (page 42) for 5 to 10 minutes.

A Minimalist's Dream

A sequence with one simple prop setup • 40 to 60 minutes

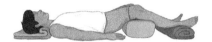

Basic Relaxation Pose

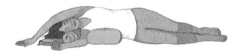

Simple Supported Side Bend

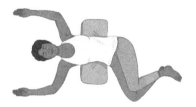

Supported Open Twist

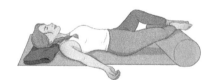

Reclining Butterfly with Feet on
the Bolster

PROPS	POSES
• Bolster (or 2 rolled blankets or a large pillow) • Blanket roll • Square eighth-fold blanket (or neck pillow)	• Basic Relaxation Pose (page 26) • Simple Supported Side Bend (page 28) • Supported Open Twist (page 48) • Reclining Butterfly with Feet on the Bolster (page 58)

- If you have a spinal injury, substitute 2 long eighth-fold blankets for the bolster in Simple Supported Side Bend and Supported Open Twist.

BENEFITS

- One sweet and simple prop setup allows you to do less and relax more.
- Gently softens the muscles of your spine and hips to promote soothing states of ease and relaxation.

TIP

In Reclining Butterfly with Feet on the Bolster, take 6 to 8 rounds of Balanced Breath as outlined on page 148 in Chapter 8 to center and calm your mind.

INSTRUCTIONS

1. Begin with 20 to 30 minutes in **Basic Relaxation Pose**, then bend your knees and roll to your side.
2. Press yourself up to a sitting position, then move your legs off to the left and move your right hip up to the edge of the bolster and tuck your feet in behind you. Guide yourself into **Simple Supported Side Bend**, for 3 to 5 minutes.
3. From **Simple Supported Side Bend**, on the right side, move directly into **Supported Open Twist** for 3 to 5 minutes.
4. Return to **Simple Supported Side Bend**, then press yourself up, leave your bolster where it is, and turn around to repeat both poses on the left side.
5. After you've completed **Supported Open Twist** on your left side, press yourself up and turn to face the bolster. Lie back and bring your feet onto the bolster to complete your practice with 5 to 8 minutes in **Reclining Butterfly with Feet on the Bolster**.

Flow Like a River

A sequence to move your spine • 45 to 70 minutes

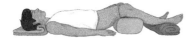

Basic Relaxation Pose

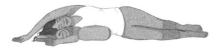

Simple Supported Side Bend

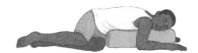

Grounding Spinal Twist

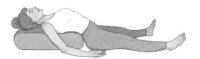

Heart Pose

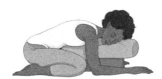

Supported Child's Pose

PROPS	POSES
• Bolster (or 2 rolled blankets or a large pillow)	• Basic Relaxation Pose (page 26)
• Blanket roll	• Simple Supported Side Bend (page 28)
• Square eighth-fold blanket (or neck pillow)	• Grounding Spinal Twist (page 30)
• 2 blocks (or large hardcover books)	• Heart Pose (page 34)
	• Supported Child's Pose (page 38)

- If you experience lower back pain or discomfort in Heart Pose, substitute Supported Heart Pose with Legs Over a Bolster (page 66).
- If Supported Child's Pose hurts your knees, substitute Supported Forward Fold (page 36).

BENEFITS

- Supports and sustains the natural mobility of your spine.
- Maintains freedom in your movements.
- Improves respiration.
- Promotes energetic states of fluidity and ease.

TIP

Use the River Meditation outlined on page 152 in Chapter 8 during Basic Relaxation Pose and enhance the sensations of ease and fluidity in your spine.

INSTRUCTIONS

1. Begin with 20 to 30 minutes in **Basic Relaxation Pose**, then bend your knees and roll to your side.
2. Press yourself up to a sitting position, then move your legs off the bolster to the left and bring your right hip up to the edge of the bolster and tuck your feet in behind you. Guide yourself into **Simple Supported Side Bend** for 3 to 5 minutes.
3. Leave your props as they are and turn yourself around to repeat the pose on the other side. After you've completed both sides, press yourself up and turn the bolster so it's lengthwise with the narrow end touching your left hip. Guide yourself into **Grounding Spinal Twist** for 3 to 5 minutes.
4. Leave your props as they are and turn yourself around to repeat the pose on the other side. After you've completed both sides, press yourself up, leave your bolster where it is, and come to a sitting position with the base of your spine touching the narrow end of the bolster and your legs extended. Guide yourself into **Heart Pose** for 5 to 10 minutes.
5. Bend your knees, roll to one side, and press yourself up to a sitting position. Turn around to face your bolster and come to your hands and knees. Prop your bolster up on the blocks and guide yourself into **Supported Child's Pose** for 5 to 8 minutes to complete your practice.

A Grateful Heart

A sequence of backbends to open your heart • 35 to 60 minutes

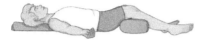

Spine Lengthening Pose

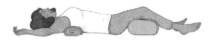

Mountain Brook

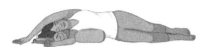

Simple Supported Side Bend

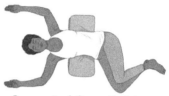

Supported Open Twist

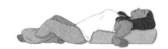

Heart Pose with Butterfly Legs

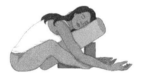

Seated Butterfly

PROPS	POSES
• Blanket roll	• Spine Lengthening Pose (page 32)
• Bolster (or 2 rolled blankets or	• Mountain Brook (page 46)
• A large pillow)	• Simple Supported Side Bend (page 28)
• Square eighth-fold blanket (or neck pillow)	• Supported Open Twist (page 48)
• 2 blocks (or large hardcover books)	• Heart Pose with Butterfly Legs (page 50)
	• Seated Butterfly (page 74)

- If you experience sensitivity in your spine with backbends, skip Heart Pose with Butterfly Legs or substitute Pregnant Goddess Pose (page 86).

BENEFITS
- Helps reverse the effects of sitting for long periods
- Encourages heart-centered emotions of love, joy, compassion, and gratitude.

TIP

Use the Gratitude Meditation outlined on page 151 during Heart Pose with Butterfly Legs and feel your heart, body, and mind opening to the flow of abundance.

INSTRUCTIONS

1. Begin with 5 to 10 minutes in **Spine Lengthening Pose**, then bend your knees and roll to your side.
2. Press yourself up to a sitting position, then adjust the blanket roll behind you so that it runs horizontally across your mat. Lie back down for 5 to 10 minutes in **Mountain Brook**.
3. Bend your knees, roll to your side, and press yourself up to a sitting position. Move your legs off the bolster to the left and bring your right hip up to the edge of the bolster and tuck your feet in behind you. Guide yourself into **Simple Supported Side Bend** for 3 to 5 minutes.
4. From **Simple Supported Side Bend** on the right side, move directly into **Supported Open Twist** for 3 to 5 minutes.
5. Return to **Simple Supported Side Bend** then press yourself up and leave your props as they are, turning yourself around to sit on the left hip and repeat both poses on the left side.
6. After you've completed both sides, press yourself up, turn your bolster so it's lengthwise, and turn yourself around to a sitting position with the base of your spine touching the narrow end of the bolster. Use your blanket roll to support your legs in a butterfly position and guide yourself into **Heart Pose with Butterfly Legs** for 5 to 10 minutes.
7. Draw your knees together, roll to one side, and press yourself up to a sitting position. Turn around to face your bolster, prop it up on the blocks, and complete your practice with 5 to 8 minutes in **Seated Butterfly**.

Inward Bound

A sequence of grounding forward bends • 45 to 60 minutes

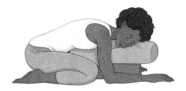

Supported Child's Pose

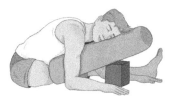

Seated Half Butterfly

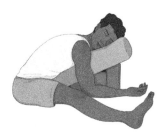

Supported Straddle Forward Fold

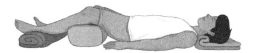

Basic Relaxation Pose

PROPS	POSES
• 2 blocks (or large hardcover books) • Bolster (or 2 rolled blankets or a large pillow) • Blanket roll • Square eighth-fold blanket (or neck pillow)	• Supported Child's Pose (page 38) • Seated Half Butterfly (page 72) • Supported Straddle Forward Fold (page 54) • Basic Relaxation Pose (page 26)

- If forward bending your spine is contraindicated, skip this sequence.
- If Supported Child's Pose hurts your knees, substitute Head to Bolster Pose (page 76).
- If Supported Straddle Forward Fold challenges your hamstrings, bend your knees a little and slide rolled-up blankets or towels beneath them.

TIP

In Basic Relaxation Pose, practice 6 to 8 rounds of Incremental Breath (page 149) and use the pauses to support your introspective journey.

BENEFITS

- Supports your spine in gentle flexion.
- Promotes states of introspection and contemplation.
- Calms and grounds your body and mind.

INSTRUCTIONS

1. Begin with 5 to 8 minutes in **Supported Child's Pose**.
2. Press yourself up to hands and knees and turn the farthest block up to its tallest setting under the bolster.
3. Move onto your seat and guide yourself into **Seated Half Butterfly** for 5 minutes on both sides.
4. Leave the bolster as it is and take your legs out long and wide for 5 to 8 minutes in **Supported Straddle Forward Fold**.
5. Press your hands into the bolster to come up. Move the blocks aside and turn your bolster so it's horizontal across your mat. Place your legs over the bolster and complete your practice with 20 to 30 minutes in **Basic Relaxation Pose**.

Nourish the Roots

A sequence for opening all four sides of your hips
20 to 30 minutes

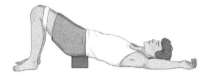

Supported Bridge

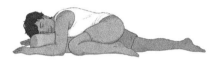

Supported Pigeon

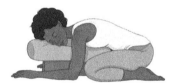

Supported Child's Pose

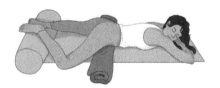

Restorative Frog

PROPS	POSES
• Yoga Strap	• Supported Bridge (page 90)
• 2 blocks (or large hardcover books)	• Supported Pigeon (page 78)
• Bolster (or 2 rolled blankets or a large pillow)	• Supported Child's Pose (page 38)
• Blanket roll	• Restorative Frog (page 60)

- If you experience knee pain in Supported Child's Pose, substitute Supported Forward Fold (page 36).
- If you experience pain or discomfort in Restorative Frog, substitute Reclining Butterfly (page 40).

BENEFITS

- Relieves tension in your hips that comes from long periods spent sitting or standing, and excessive exercise.
- Supports the natural mobility of your hips to cultivate freedom in your movements.
- Promotes earthy energetic states of surrender and renewal.

TIP

Use this sequence as part of your recovery from athletic training, which tends to strengthen your hips in only one movement pattern.

INSTRUCTIONS

1. Begin with 3 to 5 minutes in **Supported Bridge**. First, secure the yoga strap around your thighs, then lie on your back with your knees bent and your feet on the ground. Lift your hips up, placing the block on its lowest setting underneath your sacrum. Take your arms wide and relax.
2. To come out of this pose, remove the block, lower your hips, and remove the yoga strap. Roll to one side and press yourself up to your hands and knees. Arrange your bolster lengthwise in front of you and guide yourself into **Supported Pigeon** for 3 to 5 minutes on each side.
3. Come to your hands and knees and prop the bolster up on the blocks for 5 to 8 minutes in **Supported Child's Pose**.
4. Press up to hands and knees and turn the bolster so it's horizontal across your mat. Turn yourself around so the bolster is behind you, lay the blanket roll in front of you, and guide yourself into **Restorative Frog** for 3 to 5 minutes to complete your practice.

Back to Bliss

A sequence for back pain relief • 50 to 65 minutes

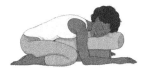

Supported Child's Pose

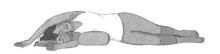

Simple Supported Side Bend

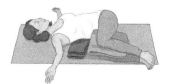

Gentle Open Twist

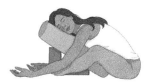

Seated Half Butterfly

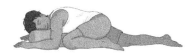

Supported Pigeon

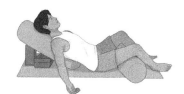

Supported Heart Pose with Legs
over a Bolster

PROPS	POSES
• 2 bolsters (or make 2 from 4 rolled blankets or 2 large pillows) • 2 blocks (or large hardcover books) • Square eighth-fold blanket • 2 long eighth-fold blankets	• Supported Child's Pose (page 38) • Simple Supported Side Bend (page 28) • Gentle Open Twist (page 68) • Seated Half Butterfly (page 72) • Supported Pigeon (page 78) • Supported Heart Pose with Legs over a Bolster (page 66)

- This is intended to be a general sequence to alleviate nonspecific back pain. If any of the poses worsen your symptoms, skip them.
- For sciatic pain, use the Sciatica S.O.S. sequence (page 120).

Enhance this sequence by finishing with Seated Meditation Pose using any of the meditation practices outlined in Chapter 8 (page 147).

BENEFITS

- Stretches muscles that can contribute to back pain when stiff.
- Gently moves your spine to relieve pressure and maintain mobility.
- Helps reduce the risk of incapacity from back pain.

INSTRUCTIONS

1. Begin with 5 to 8 minutes in **Supported Child's Pose**.
2. Press up to your hands and knees, set the blocks aside, and turn the bolster so it's horizontal across your mat. Sit on your right hip with your thigh running along the edge of the bolster. Guide yourself into **Simple Supported Side Bend** for 3 to 5 minutes. Leave the bolster where it is and turn yourself around to repeat the pose on the other side.
3. After you've completed both sides, press yourself up and exchange the bolster for 2 stacked long eighth-fold blankets. Guide yourself into **Gentle Open Twist** for 3 to 5 minutes. Leave your props as they are and turn yourself around to repeat the pose on the other side.
4. After completing both sides, press yourself up to sitting and arrange your bolster on a block for **Seated Half Butterfly**. You may choose to sit on the edge of your stacked blankets. Guide yourself through 5 minutes on each side.
5. After you've completed both sides, remove the block from under the bolster then move to your hands and knees facing the bolster, 3 to 5 minutes in **Supported Pigeon**.
6. After you've completed both sides, press yourself up and prop the bolster up on 2 blocks in preparation for **Supported Heart Pose with Legs Over a Bolster**. Come to a sitting position facing away from the bolster so the narrow end is touching the base of your spine. Place your legs over the second bolster and lie on the bolster behind you. Stay here for up to 20 minutes to complete your practice.

Sciatica S.O.S.

A sequence for sciatic pain and piriformis syndrome relief
40 to 60 minutes

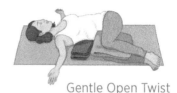

Single Leg up the Chair

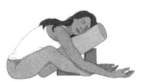

Gentle Open Twist

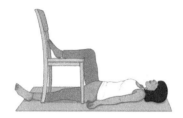

Supported Pigeon

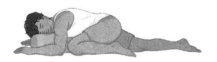

Seated Butterfly

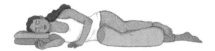

Side Lying Pose

PROPS	POSES
• Chair	• Single Leg up the Chair (page 98)
• Bolster (or 2 rolled blankets or a large pillow)	• Gentle Open Twist (page 68)
• 2 long eighth-fold blankets	• Supported Pigeon (page 78)
• 2 square eighth-fold blankets	• Seated Butterfly (page 74)
• 2 blocks (or large hardcover books)	• Side Lying Pose (page 88)

PRECAUTIONS

- Not all sciatic pain is the same. Skip any poses that increase your discomfort.
- If lying on one side worsens your symptoms, only do Side Lying Pose on the side that alleviates your symptoms.

BENEFITS

- Helps relieve sciatic pain by gently stretching the piriformis muscle, relieving pressure from your spine, and improving pelvic alignment.

TIP

If you're short on time and experiencing discomfort, do Supported Pigeon daily as it is likely the most effective pose for quick relief.

INSTRUCTIONS

1. Begin with **Single Leg up the Chair**. Do both sides for 5 to 7 minutes each.
2. Press yourself up to a sitting position and move the chair out of your way.
3. Stack your 2 long eighth-fold blankets in front of you and guide yourself into 3 to 5 minutes in **Gentle Open Twist**, placing the square eighth-fold blanket between your knees for comfort.
4. Leave the long eighth-fold blankets as they are and turn yourself around to repeat the pose on the other side, repositioning the square eighth-fold blanket accordingly. After you've completed both sides, press yourself up to a sitting position, move the blankets aside, and move to your hands and knees facing your bolster for 3 to 5 minutes in **Supported Pigeon**.
5. After you've completed both sides, press yourself up to hands and knees, arrange your bolster on a block, and come to a seated position for **Seated Butterfly** for 5 to 8 minutes.
6. Complete your practice with 5 to 8 minutes in **Side Lying Pose**.

Dissolve and Evolve

A sequence for headache, neck, and jaw tension
45 to 65 minutes

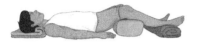

Basic Relaxation Pose

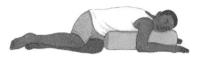

Grounding Spinal Twist

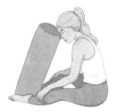

Head to Bolster Pose

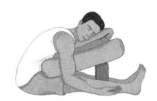

Supported Forward Fold

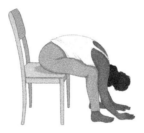

Chair Forward Fold

PROPS	POSES
• Bolster (or two rolled blankets or a large pillow) • Blanket roll • Block (or large hardcover book) • Square eighth-fold blanket (or neck pillow) • Chair	• Basic Relaxation Pose (page 26) • Grounding Spinal Twist (page 30) • Head to Bolster Pose (page 76) • Supported Forward Fold (page 36) • Chair Forward Fold (page 96)

- Inverting is contraindicated for pregnancy, hernia, severe acid reflux, brain injuries, glaucoma, and high blood pressure. If you suffer from any of these conditions, skip Chair Forward Fold.

BENEFITS

- Helps relieve generalized head, neck, and jaw pain and tension by supporting the weight of your head and encouraging your neck and jaw to relax.

TIP

In Grounding Spinal Twist, when you are sitting on your right hip, try placing your left cheek on the bolster to relieve neck tension. When you are sitting on your left hip, place your right cheek on the bolster.

INSTRUCTIONS

1. Begin with 20 to 30 minutes in **Basic Relaxation Pose**, then bend your knees and roll to your side.
2. Press yourself up to a sitting position, then move your legs off the bolster to the left so you are sitting on your right hip.
3. Turn the bolster so it's lengthwise, with the narrow end touching your right hip, then guide yourself into **Grounding Spinal Twist** for 3 to 5 minutes. Leave the bolster as it is and turn your body around to repeat the pose on the other side.
4. After you've completed both sides, press yourself up to a sitting position facing the bolster and move into **Head to Bolster Pose** for 5 to 8 minutes.
5. Press yourself up and prop your bolster on the block topped with the square eighth-fold blanket and relax for 5 to 8 minutes in **Supported Forward Fold**.
6. Finally, move to a chair for 3 to 5 minutes in **Chair Forward Fold**.

Air Becomes Breath

A soothing sequence for asthma • 45 to 75 minutes

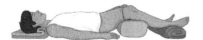

Basic Relaxation Pose

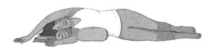

Simple Supported Side Bend

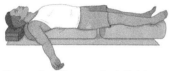

Extended Supported Bridge

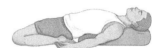

Reclining Hero Pose

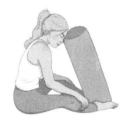

Head to Bolster Pose

PROPS	POSES
• 2 bolsters (or make 2 from 4 rolled blankets or 2 large pillows) • Blanket roll • Block (or large hardcover book) • Square eighth-fold blanket	• Basic Relaxation Pose (page 26) • Simple Supported Side Bend (page 28) • Extended Supported Bridge (page 52) • Reclining Hero Pose (page 92) • Head to Bolster Pose (page 76)

- If Reclining Hero Pose is not suitable for your knees or lower back, substitute Heart Pose (page 34).

BENEFITS

- Reduces stress and anxiety.
- Creates space in your chest and lungs to facilitate healthy breathing.

TIP

After you've completely relaxed in Basic Relaxation Pose, begin Spinal Breath as described in Chapter 8 (page 147).

INSTRUCTIONS

1. Begin with 20 to 30 minutes in **Basic Relaxation Pose**, then bend your knees and roll to your side.
2. Press yourself up to a sitting position, then move your legs off the bolster to the left so you are sitting on your right hip with your right thigh running along the edge of the bolster and your feet tucked in behind you. Guide yourself into **Simple Supported Side Bend** for 3 to 5 minutes. Leave your bolster as it is and turn yourself around to repeat the pose on the other side.
3. Press yourself up to a sitting position, then place the two bolsters end to end with the block at one end for your head. Guide yourself into **Extended Supported Bridge** for 8 to 10 minutes.
4. Carefully roll off the bolsters and press yourself up to a sitting position. Move one of the bolsters aside and come to kneeling with the bolster behind you for 3 to 5 minutes in **Reclining Hero Pose**.
5. Press yourself up to a sitting position, turn to face the bolster with your legs outstretched, and complete your practice with 5 to 8 minutes in **Head to Bolster Pose**.

Unwind and Recharge

A sequence for stress and fatigue • 45 to 75 minutes

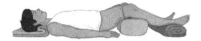

Basic Relaxation Pose

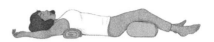

Mountain Brook

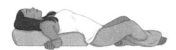

Heart Pose with Butterfly Legs

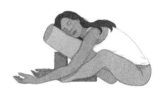

Seated Butterfly

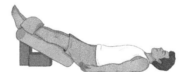

Legs Up the Bolster

PROPS	POSES
• Bolster (or 2 rolled blankets or a large pillow) • Blanket roll • Square eighth-fold blanket (or neck pillow) • 2 blocks (or large hardcover books) • Sandbag (or heavy folded blanket)	• Basic Relaxation Pose (page 26) • Mountain Brook (page 46) • Heart Pose with Butterfly Legs (page 50) • Seated Butterfly (page 74) • Legs Up the Bolster (page 82)

- If you experience lower back pain or discomfort in Heart Pose with Butterfly Legs, substitute Pregnant Goddess Pose (page 86).

BENEFITS

- Relaxes and supports your entire body.
- Gently opens your hips and heart.
- Brings awareness to your breath.
- Promotes vitality.

TIP

Deep breathing exercises and visualization have proven to be highly effective in managing stress and fatigue. In Basic Relaxation Pose, employ the Body Scan Meditation and Spinal Breath described in Chapter 8 (page 147).

INSTRUCTIONS

1. Begin with 20 to 30 minutes in **Basic Relaxation Pose**, then bend your knees and roll to your side.
2. Press yourself up to a sitting position. Take the blanket roll out from underneath your ankles and place it behind your upper back for 5 to 10 minutes in **Mountain Brook**.
3. Bend your knees and roll to your side. Press yourself up to a sitting position, then turn the bolster so it's lengthwise. Turn yourself around so the narrow end of the bolster is touching the base of your spine. Use the blanket roll from **Mountain Brook** to secure your legs in a butterfly position, then lie back for 5 to 10 minutes in **Heart Pose with Butterfly Legs**.
4. Draw your knees together, roll to your side, and press yourself up to a sitting position. Turn around to face the bolster, prop it up on your blocks, and guide yourself into **Seated Butterfly** for 5 to 8 minutes.
5. Bring your legs up the bolster and lie back for 5 to 10 minutes in **Legs Up the Bolster** to complete your practice.

Steady as You Go

A sequence to ease anxiety • 35 to 55 minutes

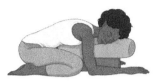

Supported Child's Pose

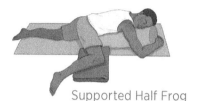

Supported Half Frog

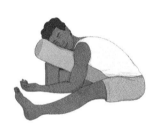

Supported Straddle Forward Fold

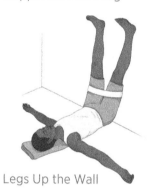

Legs Up the Wall

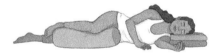

Side Lying Pose

PROPS	POSES
• Bolster (or 2 rolled blankets or a large pillow) • Long eighth-fold blanket • 2 blocks (or large hardcover books) • Yoga strap • 2 square eighth-fold blanket	• Supported Child's Pose (page 38) • Supported Half Frog (page 80) • Supported Straddle Forward Fold (page 54) • Legs Up the Wall (page 62) • Side Lying Pose (page 88)

- If you experience knee pain in Supported Child's Pose, substitute Restorative Frog (page 60).
- Inverting is contraindicated for pregnancy, hernia, severe acid reflux, brain injuries, glaucoma, and high blood pressure. If you suffer from any of these conditions, skip Legs Up the Wall.

TIP

In this practice, lengthen your exhales to help slow your heart rate and cultivate the relaxation response.

BENEFITS

- Supports your body and calms your mind.
- Draws energy and awareness down into the roots of your body.
- Cultivates states of grounding and stability to combat the stimulation of anxiety.

INSTRUCTIONS

1. Set up your mat so the narrow end is touching the wall.
2. Begin with 5 to 8 minutes in **Supported Child's Pose**.
3. Press up to hands and knees and guide yourself into **Supported Half Frog** for 3 to 5 minutes on each side.
4. After you've completed both sides, press yourself up to hands and knees and come to a sitting position with your legs out long and wide on either side of the bolster. Prop your bolster up onto the blocks and guide yourself into **Supported Straddle Forward Fold** for 5 to 8 minutes.
5. Move the bolster and blocks out of your way, move to the wall, secure the yoga strap around your thighs, and spend 5 to 10 minutes in **Legs Up the Wall**.
6. Bend your knees and roll onto one side. Press yourself up to a sitting position, then arrange your bolster and blankets to complete your practice with 5 to 10 minutes on each side in **Side Lying Pose**.

Let Your Soul Shine

A sequence to ease grief and depression • 40 to 60 minutes

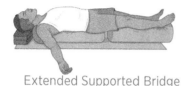

Extended Supported Bridge

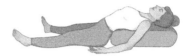

Heart Pose

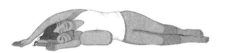

Simple Supported Side Bend

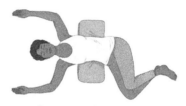

Supported Open Twist

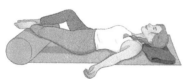

Reclining Butterfly with Feet
on the Bolster

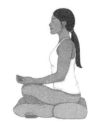

Seated Meditation Pose

PROPS	POSES
• 2 bolsters (or make 2 from 4 rolled blankets or 2 large pillows) • Block (or large hardcover book) • Blanket roll • Square eighth-fold blanket	• Extended Supported Bridge (page 52) • Heart Pose (page 34) • Simple Supported Side Bend (page 28) • Supported Open Twist (page 48) • Reclining Butterfly with Feet on the Bolster (page 58) • Seated Meditation Pose (page 102)

- If you experience lower back pain or discomfort in Heart Pose, skip it.

BENEFITS

- Cultivates uplifting sensations of space and opening to counter the heaviness of grief and depression.
- Focuses on opening your heart to promote feelings
of love, joy, compassion, and gratitude.

TIP

In Seated Meditation Pose, use the Loving-Kindness Meditation outlined in Chapter 8 (page 147) to cultivate feelings of abundance and connection.

INSTRUCTIONS

1. Position your bolsters and block and begin with 8 to 10 minutes in **Extended Supported Bridge**.
2. Carefully roll off the bolsters and press yourself up to a sitting position. Move one bolster aside and sit with the base of your spine touching the narrow end of the remaining bolster. Guide yourself into **Heart Pose** for 5 to 10 minutes.
3. Bend your knees, roll to your right side, and press yourself up to sitting on your right hip. Turn the bolster so it's horizontal across your mat with the long edge running along your right thigh. Guide yourself into **Simple Supported Side Bend** for 3 to 5 minutes.
4. From **Simple Supported Side Bend** on the right side, move directly into **Supported Open Twist** for 3 to 5 minutes.
5. Return to **Simple Supported Side Bend**, then press yourself up, leave your bolster where it is, and turn around to repeat both poses on the left side.
6. After you've completed both sides, press yourself up to a sitting position. Face your bolster and lie back with the soles of your feet pressed together and resting on the bolster, for 5 to 8 minutes in **Reclining Butterfly with Feet on the Bolster**.
7. Roll to one side and press yourself up and sit on your bolster to complete your practice with 3 to 5 minutes in **Seated Meditation Pose**.

Brand New Day

A short, gentle, and energizing morning sequence
35 to 50 minutes

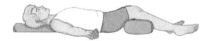

Spine Lengthening Pose

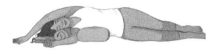

Simple Supported Side Bend

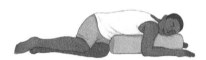

Grounding Spinal Twist

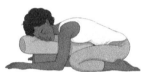

Supported Child's Pose

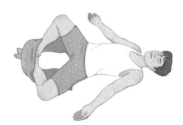

Reclining Butterfly

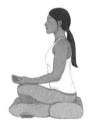

Seated Meditation Pose

PROPS	POSES
• Square eighth-fold blanket	• Spine Lengthening Pose (page 32)
• Long eighth-fold blanket	• Simple Supported Side Bend (page 28)
• Bolster (or 2 rolled blankets or a large pillow)	• Grounding Spinal Twist (page 30)
	• Supported Child's Pose (page 38)
• 2 blocks (or large hardcover books)	• Reclining Butterfly (page 40)
• Blanket roll	• Seated Meditation Pose (page 102)

- Avoid any extreme movements with your spine early in the morning as your spinal discs are at their fullest after lying down overnight for sleep, which makes your back stiffer than it is later in the day.

TIP

In Seated Medita-tion Pose, take 8 to 10 rounds of Sun Breath as described in Chapter 8 (page 147).

BENEFITS

- Gently stimulates your body and mind to flush out the heaviness of sleep.
- Prepares your body and mind for seated meditation.
- Energizes you for the day ahead.

INSTRUCTIONS

1. Begin with up to 10 minutes in **Spine Lengthening Pose**, then bend your knees and roll to your side.
2. Press yourself up to a sitting position, then move your legs off the bolster to the left so you are sitting on your right hip with your right thigh running along the edge of the bolster and your feet tucked in behind you. Guide yourself into **Simple Supported Side Bend** for 3 to 5 minutes.
3. Leave your props where they are and turn your body around to repeat the pose on the other side. After you've completed both sides, press yourself up to a sitting position and turn the bolster so it's lengthwise with the narrow end touching your left hip. Guide yourself into **Grounding Spinal Twist** for 3 to 5 minutes.
4. Leave your props where they are and turn your body around to change sides. After you've completed both sides, press yourself up to hands and knees.
5. Prop the bolster up on the blocks and take 5 to 8 minutes in **Supported Child's Pose**.
6. Press up to hands and knees and move the bolster out of your way. Come to your seat and use the blanket roll to support your legs in a butterfly position. Place the long eighth-fold blanket behind you and lie back for 5 to 8 minutes in **Reclining Butterfly**.
7. Draw your knees together and roll to your side, then press yourself up and sit on your bolster to complete your practice with 3 to 5 minutes in **Seated Meditation Pose.**

Fly Me to the Moon

A tranquil evening sequence to aid sleep • 55 to 75 minutes

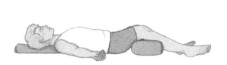

Spine Lengthening Pose

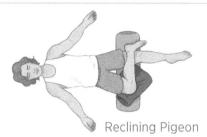

Reclining Pigeon

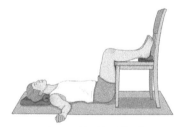

Grounding Spinal Twist

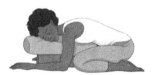

Supported Child's Pose

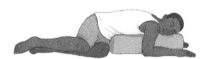

Legs Up the Chair

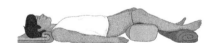

Basic Relaxation Pose

PROPS	POSES
• Bolster (or 2 rolled blankets or a large pillow)	• Spine Lengthening Pose (page 32)
• Blanket roll	• Reclining Pigeon (page 56)
• Square eighth-fold blanket (or neck pillow)	• Grounding Spinal Twist (page 30)
• 2 blocks (or large hardcover books)	• Supported Child's Pose (page 38)
• Chair	• Legs Up the Chair (page 100)
	• Basic Relaxation Pose (page 26)

- Gently stretches your spine to relieve pressure built up during the day.
- Can alleviate swollen feet and tired legs after standing and walking during the day.
- Calms your mind and relaxes your body.
- Relieves insomnia and supports deep, restful sleep.

TIP

Before or after your practice, take 8 to 10 rounds of Moon Breath as outlined in Chapter 8 (page 147) to soothe your nervous system and prepare for sleep.

INSTRUCTIONS

1. Begin with up to 10 minutes in **Spine Lengthening Pose**.
2. Bend your knees and roll to one side. Press yourself up to a sitting position and move the blanket roll from behind you.
3. Cross your right ankle over your left knee, support your right knee with a blanket, and lie back for 3 to 5 minutes in **Reclining Pigeon**. Repeat on the opposite side.
4. After you've completed both sides, bend your knees, roll onto your side, and press yourself up to a sitting position on your right hip, with your feet tucked in behind you. Turn the bolster so it's lengthwise with the narrow end touching your right hip. Guide yourself into **Grounding Spinal Twist** for 3 to 5 minutes.
5. Leave the props as they are and turn your body around to stretch the other side.
6. After you've completed both sides, press yourself up and leave the bolster as it is. Make your way onto your hands and knees and prop the bolster up on the blocks for 5 to 8 minutes in **Supported Child's Pose**.
7. Press up to hands and knees and move the bolster out of your way. Come to a sitting position near the chair and guide yourself into **Legs Up the Chair**; remain there for 5 to 10 minutes.
8. Complete your practice by rolling to one side and setting up for 20 to 30 minutes in **Basic Relaxation Pose**.

Smooth Cycle

**A sequence for menstrual pain and discomfort
60 to 80 minutes**

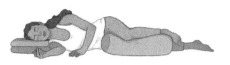

Side Lying Pose

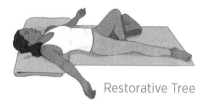

Restorative Tree

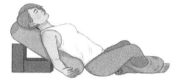

Pregnant Goddess Pose

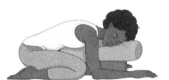

Supported Child's Pose

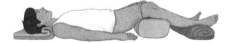

Basic Relaxation Pose

PROPS	POSES
• Bolster (or 2 rolled blankets or a large pillow) • Quarter-fold blanket • 2 square eighth-fold blankets • Blanket roll • 2 blocks (or large hardcover books)	• Side Lying Pose (page 88) • Restorative Tree (page 70) • Pregnant Goddess Pose (page 86) • Supported Child's Pose (page 38) • Basic Relaxation Pose (page 26)

- If Supported Child's Pose hurts your knees, substitute Seated Butterfly (page 74).

BENEFITS

- Eases pain and discomfort before and during your menstrual cycle.
- Elicits much needed rest during menstruation.

INSTRUCTIONS

1. Begin with 5 to 10 minutes per side in **Side Lying Pose**.
2. After you've completed both sides, press yourself up to a sitting position and move the bolster aside. Lie back and guide yourself into **Restorative Tree** for 5 minutes per side.
3. After you've completed both sides, bend your knees, roll onto one side, and press yourself up to a sitting position. Stack the bolster on the L-shape positioned blocks. Turn yourself around so the narrow end is touching the base of your spine, use the blanket roll to support your legs in a butterfly position and lie back onto the bolster for 8 to 12 minutes in **Pregnant Goddess Pose**.
4. Draw your knees together and roll to one side. Press yourself up to a sitting position, then turn to face your bolster, coming onto hands and knees. Ensure the blocks under the bolster are now the same height and guide yourself into **Supported Child's Pose** for 5 to 8 minutes.
5. Press yourself up to hands and knees, remove the blocks and turn the bolster so it's horizontal across your mat. Come into a sitting position with your legs over the bolster and lie back to complete your practice with 20 to 30 minutes in **Basic Relaxation Pose**.

Family Style

A short sequence you can enjoy with the kids • 20 minutes

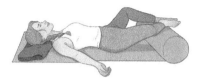

Reclining Butterfly with Feet
on the Bolster

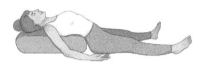

Heart Pose

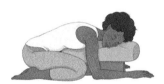

Supported Child's Pose

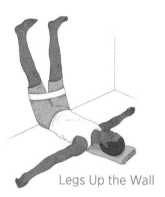

Legs Up the Wall

PROPS	POSES
• Bolster (or 2 rolled blankets or a large pillow) for each person • Square eighth-fold blanket for each person • 2 blocks for each person	• Reclining Butterfly with Feet on the Bolster (page 58) • Heart Pose (page 34) • Supported Child's Pose (page 38) • Legs Up the Wall (page 62)

- For young children under the age of 10, substitute a folded blanket or a pillow for the bolster to ensure comfort.

BENEFITS

- Encourages healthy quality time together with your family.
- Yoga can help your child develop focus and self-esteem, and reduce stress and anxiety.

INSTRUCTIONS

1. Set up your mats so that the narrow end is close to the wall. Leave about a foot of space between each mat if possible.
2. Begin with 5 minutes in **Reclining Butterfly with Feet on the Bolster**.
3. Draw your knees together and roll to one side. Press yourself up and turn the bolster so it's vertical on your mat. Turn around so the narrow end touches the base of your spine and lie back for 5 minutes in **Heart Pose**.
4. Bend your knees, roll to one side and press yourself up to a sitting position. Move onto your hands and knees facing the bolster and prop it up onto the blocks, then guide yourself into **Supported Child's Pose** for 5 minutes.
5. Press up to your hands and knees, move the bolster aside, and come to the wall to complete your practice with 5 minutes in **Legs Up the Wall**. You can do this pose without the strap to make things less complicated—simply lie back and bring your legs up the wall.

Office Space

A sequence to break up the workday • 20 minutes

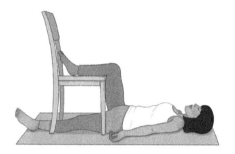

Single Leg Up the Chair

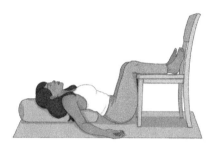

Heart Pose with a Chair

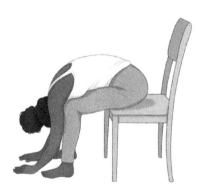

Chair Forward Fold

PROPS	POSES
• Chair • Bolster (or 2 rolled blankets or a large pillow)	• Single Leg Up the Chair (page 98) • Heart Pose with a Chair (page 94) • Chair Forward Fold (page 96)

- Inverting is contraindicated for pregnancy, hernia, severe acid reflux, brain injuries, glaucoma, and high blood pressure. If you suffer from any of these conditions, skip Chair Forward Fold.

BENEFITS
- A short and sweet practice with minimal props that can relieve the effects of extended periods spent sitting, such as tension in your hips, neck, and jaw.

INSTRUCTIONS

1. Start by doing **Single Leg Up the Chair** for 5 minutes on each side.
2. Roll to one side and press up to a sitting position. Arrange your bolster behind you so the narrow end touches the base of your spine. Bring both legs back up onto the chair for 5 minutes in **Heart Pose with a Chair**.
3. Roll carefully to one side, then press yourself up to a sitting position. After a moment, sit up on the chair and complete your practice with 3 minutes in **Chair Forward Fold**.

Mindful Mama

A safe and satisfying sequence for pregnancy • 30 to 40 minutes

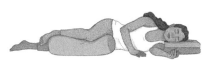

Side Lying Pose

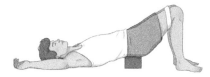

Supported Bridge

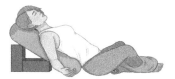

Pregnant Goddess Pose

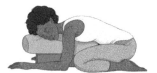

Supported Child's Pose

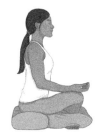

Seated Meditation

PROPS	POSES
• Bolster (or 2 rolled blankets or a large pillow)	• Side Lying Pose (left side only; page 88)
• 2 square eighth-fold blankets	• Supported Bridge (page 90)
• Yoga strap	• Pregnant Goddess Pose (page 86)
• 2 blocks (or large hardcover books)	• Supported Child's Pose (page 38)
• Blanket roll	• Seated Meditation (page 102)

- Only take Side Lying Pose on your left side during pregnancy to avoid compression of the inferior vena cava. (The vena cava is an important vein that runs slightly to the right side of your spine and returns the blood from your lower body to your heart. As your pregnancy progresses, the weight of the baby and your increased blood volume can inhibit this blood flow when you lie on your right side.)
- This sequence is generally appropriate during all three trimesters; however, as your pregnancy progresses, if any pose becomes uncomfortable, skip it.
- Toward the end of your pregnancy, you may need to slide a square eighth-fold blanket or two underneath your belly for extra support in Supported Child's Pose.

TIP

Use your practice at this time to cultivate Spinal Breath, as described in Chapter 8 (page 147). This calming breath helps prepare women for labor.

BENEFITS

- Creates a safe and supported space for much-needed rest and relaxation during your pregnancy.
- Gently opens your hips to relieve lower back pain and prepare for childbirth.
- Fosters states of awareness and mindfulness during this transformative time.

Continued >

continued from page 143

INSTRUCTIONS

1. Begin with 5 to 10 minutes in **Side Lying Pose** on your left side.
2. Move the bolster aside and roll onto your back. Place the yoga strap around your thighs and the block under your hips for **Supported Bridge**; remain here for 3 minutes.
3. Remove the block and yoga strap and roll to your left side, then press yourself up to a sitting position. Set up your bolster on the blocks and sit with the base of your spine touching the end of the bolster. Use the blanket roll to support your legs in a butterfly position. Guide yourself into **Pregnant Goddess Pose** and remain here for 8 to 12 minutes.
4. Draw your knees together and roll to your left side. Press yourself up and come to hands and knees facing the bolster. Prop the bolster up on the blocks for 5 to 8 minutes in **Supported Child's Pose**. As your pregnancy progresses, you may have to slide the bolster forward and take your knees wider to make room for your baby.
5. Press yourself up to hands and knees then sit on the bolster to complete your practice with 3 to 5 minutes in **Seated Meditation Pose**.

Build Your Own Sequence

These are some tips for where to start when building your own sequence. Remember, you can't do this wrong.

- Start with **Basic Relaxation Pose** (page 26) and a **Body Scan** meditation (page 151).
- Aim to include about 4 to 6 poses total.
- If you spend a lot of the day sitting, make sure to include a backbend, a side bend, and a twist to relieve pressure on your spine.
- If you're feeling down, tired, or heavy, include **Simple Supported Side Bend** (page 28) and follow it with at least one backbend, such as **Spine Lengthening Pose** (page 32), **Mountain Brook** (page 46), or a variation of **Heart Pose** (page 34).
- If you're feeling anxious, scattered, or restless, include at least one forward bend, such as **Supported Child's Pose** (page 38), **Supported Forward Fold** (page 36), or **Supported Straddle Forward Fold** (page 54), and follow it with a grounding hip opener, such as **Supported Pigeon** (page 78) or **Reclining Butterfly** (page 40).
- Generally, try to end your practice with a grounding pose, such as a forward fold, an inversion, **Seated Meditation Pose** (page 102), **Side Lying Pose** (page 88), or even **Basic Relaxation Pose** (page 26) again.
- Don't be afraid to color outside the lines and experiment with what feels good to you.
- Most important: Always include your favorite pose!

CHAPTER 8

Breathing and Meditations

Practices to control the flow of breath abound in yoga tradition as a means to conserve *prana*, vital energy, which we receive via the breath. In scientific terms, controlling the breath is a means to access and control the unconscious functions of the autonomic nervous system, such as digestion, heart rate, and the stress and relaxation responses. There are countless breathing exercises in the yoga tradition, and the ones included here are very gentle, simple techniques appropriate for beginners and for restorative yoga.

Breathing Exercises

You may choose one or two techniques each time you practice. These can be done sitting in Seated Meditation Pose (page 102), or lying in Basic Relaxation Pose (page 26) or Spine Lengthening Pose (page 32). Always give your body and breath time to completely relax before beginning a breathing exercise. Remember, you should never experience any strain with these techniques.

Balanced Breath

Balanced Breath is a simple practice that creates the sensation of receiving and giving in equal measure, eliminating any energetic deficit.

1. Bring your awareness to your breath and, for a few cycles, simply notice the natural length of your inhale and exhale. Don't try to modify your breath yet.
2. Begin to breathe in for approximately 4 seconds, and breathe out for 4 seconds so your inhale and exhale are equal in length. If 4 seconds feels either too long or too rushed, modify the length, but ensure that the inhale and exhale remain equal in length. There should be no strain.
3. Take 6 to 8 rounds of Balanced Breath and, when complete, return to regular, effortless breathing.
4. Observe any shifts in your breath and energy that may come from balancing effort with release.

Spinal Breath

Spinal Breath is an effective way to lengthen your breath without strain or force and draw awareness to the center of your body.

1. Bring your awareness to your breath and simply observe its natural length and depth for a few cycles.
2. Begin to imagine you are inhaling all the way down to the base of your spine and exhaling from the base all the way up your spine to the crown of your head. Do this without strain.
3. Imagine your spine growing longer with each inhale. Feel it softening with each exhale.
4. After 8 to 10 rounds, return your breathing to normal and observe any new sensations of length or depth in your body and breath.

Incremental Breath

Incremental Breath uses short, gentle pauses within your inhale to create opportunity for self-reflection and participation with your breath.

1. Bring your awareness to your breath and observe its natural flow, without trying to change it. Let it breathe you.
2. To begin Incremental Breath, take a complete exhale, then take about one-third of a breath in and briefly pause for 1 to 2 seconds. Inhale another third and pause. Finally inhale to the top of your breath and pause. Exhale all the way out, without pausing, then begin again. It is helpful to visualize a well, slowly filling with water, then emptying.
3. Take 6 to 8 rounds of Incremental Breath. Ensure that you do not, at any time, hold your breath to the point of strain or discomfort; rather, this should feel as though you are gently sipping your breath. There should be no gasping.
4. When you are finished, return your breathing to normal and observe how smooth and easy it feels now.

Sun Breath

Sun Breath focuses on opening the solar energy channel, which is described in several ancient yoga texts as flowing between the right sit bone and the right nostril. Facilitating the free flow of energy through this channel is believed to activate vitality, productivity, and strength.

1. From a comfortable seated position, bring your awareness to your breath. Take a few easy breaths.
2. Use your left thumb to gently seal your left nostril and begin to breathe in and out only through your right nostril. Your breath should be gentle.
3. Take 8 to 10 breaths, then release your hand into your lap and let your breathing return to normal.
4. Visualize an energy channel running up your spine from your right sit bone to your right nostril and feel the flow of energy between those two points. Observe any sensations of clarity and lightness in your mind.
5. For a gentler alternative to Sun Breath, use your imagination to breathe only through your right nostril while lying in Basic Relaxation Pose (page 26).

Moon Breath

Moon Breath focuses on opening the lunar energy channel, which is described in several ancient yoga texts as flowing between the left sit bone and the left nostril. Facilitating the free flow of energy through this channel is believed to invite calm, receptivity, and ease.

1. From a comfortable seated position, bring your awareness to your breath. Take a few easy breaths.
2. Use your right thumb to gently seal your right nostril and begin to breathe in and out only through your left nostril. Your breath should be gentle.
3. Take 8 to 10 breaths, then release your hand into your lap and let your breathing return to normal.
4. Visualize an energy channel running up your spine from your left sit bone to your left nostril and feel the quiet flow of energy between those two points. Notice any sensations of tranquility or nourishment.
5. As an alternative to Moon Breath, use your imagination to breathe only through your left nostril while lying in Basic Relaxation Pose (page 26).

Meditations

Meditation is the practice of mastering your mind. There are many techniques from the yoga tradition designed to focus your mind, transforming distraction into attention by connecting to sources of guidance and inspiration. These can take the form of breath observation, repetition of positive affirmations, and visualizations.

Restorative yoga is, in many ways, an extended meditation practice, where you relax your body and quiet your mind, so your direct experience can become the central focus of your attention. Although there is no need to integrate a formal meditation technique into your restorative yoga practice, it can be a very effective time to do so. Provided that you give your body enough time to relax first, you can incorporate any of the meditations described here into your practice during supine postures like Basic Relaxation Pose (page 26) or Heart Pose (page 34), or use your practice to prepare your body and mind for a seated meditation at the conclusion of your practice. And although there is no "correct" amount of time to spend in meditation, 5 to 10 minutes is a great place to start.

Body Scan

The Body Scan is a practice of mindful, deep relaxation, bringing awareness to different parts of your body to calm your nervous system. You can do it at the beginning or end of your practice.

1. In Basic Relaxation Pose (page 26), feel the weight of your body against the ground. Notice each place where you come into contact with the ground and feel the support beneath you. Relax into that support.
2. Bring your awareness to the soles of your feet. Relax the soles of your feet. Bring your awareness to the tops of your feet. Relax the tops of your feet.
3. Slowly and methodically, work your way up your body, feeling each individual body part, then relaxing it. Include your legs, torso, arms, neck, and head.
4. Soften the crown of your head. Now feel your entire body from head to toe, relaxed, soft, and heavy. Notice each place where you come into contact with the ground and feel the support beneath you. Relax deeper into that support.

Gratitude Meditation

Psychology research has shown that practicing gratitude increases emotional happiness, improves health and relationships, and even helps you deal with adversity. This meditation is ideal for any time you're experiencing sadness or scarcity and can be done in Seated Meditation Pose (page 102), Basic Relaxation Pose (page 26), or any backbend posture.

1. Begin to tune in to your inner state. Observe the quality of your thoughts and emotions. Notice whether you're feeling positive and happy or negative and melancholy. Whatever your findings, please don't judge yourself.
2. Find something in your immediate physical experience to be grateful for. Let it be something simple and tangible, such as your breath, the props supporting you, or the ability of your body to do this practice. Silently say to yourself, "I am grateful for this blessing."
3. Continue identifying immediate physical blessings, from the clothes you're wearing to the roof over your head, taking a moment to truly feel and express gratitude for each item.
4. Move beyond your physical experience and identify other gifts you're in receipt of. These may include your relationships, family, profession, health, past occurrences, and present opportunities. Nothing is too small.

5. When your mind stops identifying items, hold them all in your heart and rest in the steady flow of abundance. Give thanks, then let go and turn your attention back to your breath.

River Meditation

A river is a simple but effective image from nature that reminds us of our own fluid power and malleability. This meditation is perfect for when you're feeling frustrated or stuck in life, and unsure which way to turn. It is particularly effective in Spine Lengthening Pose (page 32) and Mountain Brook (page 46).

1. Bring your awareness to your spine. Feel its natural curves from your tailbone to the small of your back, then follow it up to the back of your heart and continue to track it up to where your neck meets your head. Feel your breath softening your body the way the currents of a river soften its banks.

2. Now picture yourself sitting on the soft banks of a gentle river winding through the forest. See how easily it flows over and around rocks and trees in its path, without hesitation or struggle. Notice how when it picks up debris, such as leaves and branches, the water's flow simply washes them downstream.

3. Dip a toe into the river and feel that the water is warm and inviting. Imagine yourself safely floating down the river, joining its slow currents to carve a path through the landscape of your life. Let the currents soften your body and feel your ability to flow around obstacles placed in your path. Float downstream and feel tension dissolve from your body and worries wash away from your mind.

4. Soon, you'll come to an eddy and easily climb out of the river and lie on the bank to dry off in the sun. Return to your body and the room but continue to feel the soft reminder of currents of energy and breath flowing within you.

Ocean Meditation

Philosophers have long maintained that time spent in nature is vital for our health, and scientific research has shown that people in coastal areas tend to be happier than those inland. Many of us find the sight and sound of the ocean to be particularly healing, and this meditation is intended to recreate that healing state no matter where you are. Practice this meditation in any supine posture, or when in Seated Meditation Pose (page 102).

1. Bring your awareness to your breath. Notice how it sounds like the ocean.

2. Now imagine you are sitting on the beach, watching the ocean. Feel the sun and breeze on your skin, the soft sand underneath you. Hear the call of the birds in the sky above you and the sound of the gentle tide. Observe the waves washing up onto the shore, then gliding back into the ocean.

3. Begin to synchronize your breath with the tide. As you inhale, imagine you are drawing the waves toward you as they wash up the beach. As you exhale, send them back to join the ocean. Feel that you are not separate from the waves or the ocean.

4. Let each exhale wash away pain and sadness. Feel each inhale fill you with compassion and joy. Enjoy this breath for 3 to 5 minutes.

5. Now return to the sensations within your body and feel your breath return to normal.

Loving-Kindness Meditation

This meditation comes from the Buddhist tradition and is a powerful tool for cultivating forgiveness, goodwill, and compassion for all beings. You can practice this meditation any time, but it is particularly useful if you have unresolved conflict with others, or are experiencing feelings of envy or resentment toward others. Practice this in any supine position or Seated Meditation Pose (page 102):

1. Bring your awareness to your heart. Take a few easy breaths.

2. Keeping your awareness on yourself, silently repeat 3 times, "May I be happy. May I be healthy. May I be free."

3. Visualize someone you love very much. Hold this person's face in your mind and offer them the same good fortune: "May you be happy. May you be healthy. May you be free."

4. Now picture someone who you don't know as intimately, perhaps a neighbor or a coworker. Offer them the same intention that you easily gave to your loved one: "May you be happy. May you be healthy. May you be free."

5. Visualize yourself as a beacon of light bestowing your blessings to all beings: "May you be happy. May you be healthy. May you be free." Bask in the feeling of connection and joy that comes from offering the love in your own heart to all others.

Resources

Recommended Reading

Castle, Victoria. *The Trance of Scarcity: Stop Holding Your Breath and Start Living Your Life.* Oakland, CA: Berrett-Koehler, 2006.

Childre, D., and H. Martin. *The HeartMath Solution: The Institute of HeartMath's Revolutionary Program for Engaging the Power of the Heart's Intelligence.* San Francisco: HarperOne, 1999.

Devi, Nischala Joy. *The Healing Path of Yoga: Time-Honored Wisdom and Scientifically Proven Methods That Alleviate Stress, Open Your Heart, and Enrich Your Life.* New York: Three Rivers Press, 2000.

Lasater, Judith. *Relax and Renew: Restful Yoga for Stressful Times.* Berkeley, CA: Rodmell Press, 1995.

Pearsell, Paul. *The Heart's Code: Tapping the Wisdom and Power of Our Heart Energy.* Portland, OR: Broadway Books, 1998.

Roche, Lorin. *The Radiance Sutras: 112 Gateways to the Yoga of Wonder and Delight.* Louisville, CO: Sounds True, 2014.

Seaward, Brian. *Managing Stress: Principles and Strategies for Health and Wellbeing.* Burlington, MA: Jones & Bartlett, 2015.

Buying Yoga Props

Although you can always practice restorative yoga using items you already own, if you decide to invest in yoga props there are many good online options. For the most affordable props, I recommend either those from the Yoga Accessories or Yoga Direct websites. For high-quality props, I recommend those by Hugger Mugger and Manduka. You can refer to the list of "Nice-to-Have Props" on page 16 to decide which items to buy and determine the correct dimensions. A few notes on buying props:

Blankets

- Blankets are the most versatile prop and relatively inexpensive, so, at minimum, I recommend buying four to six yoga blankets or traditional Mexican blankets and using them to build bolsters and neck pillows.

Blocks

- Blocks are another inexpensive and versatile prop. I recommend buying two cork blocks, as these are more durable and supportive than foam blocks.

Bolsters

- Bolsters are the most expensive prop needed for restorative yoga. If you want to start with one, I recommend buying a rectangular bolster, as they are the most versatile. You may supplement this with a round bolster to go underneath your knees in many reclining postures, and a pranayama bolster, which is a slimmer bolster that can take the place of a blanket roll under your ankles in poses like Basic Relaxation Pose (page 26), and even behind your spine in Spine Lengthening Pose (page 32).

Eye Pillows

- An eye pillow is a small and relatively inexpensive prop that can make a surprisingly big difference in your ability to relax. You can find them scented or unscented; choose one according to your preference.

References

Andrews, Linda Wasmer. "Good Posture May Ease Symptoms of Depression." *Psychology Today*. January 30, 2017. www.psychologytoday.com/us/blog/minding-the-body/201701/good-posture-may-ease-symptoms-depression.

Bergland, Christopher. "Cortisol: Why the 'Stress Hormone' Is Public Enemy No. 1." *Psychology Today*. January 22, 2013. www.psychologytoday.com/us/blog/the-athletes-way/201301/cortisol-why-the-stress-hormone-is-public-enemy-no-1.

CABA. "How (and Why) to Boost Your Alpha Brainwaves." Accessed July 2, 2019. www.caba.org.uk/help-and-guides/information/how-and-why-boost-your-alpha-brainwaves.

Cheryl K. "Stress & Brain Waves." American Nutrition Association. October 31, 2009. http://americannutritionassociation.org/node/257.

Childre, D., and H. Martin. *The HeartMath Solution: The Institute of HeartMath's Revolutionary Program for Engaging the Power of the Heart's Intelligence.* San Francisco: HarperOne, 1999.

Clear, James. "How to Build a New Habit: This Is Your Strategy Guide." Accessed July 7, 2019. https://jamesclear.com/habit-guide.

Cook, Rena, and Jane Boston. *Breath in Action: The Art of Breath in Vocal and Holistic Practice.* London: Jessica Kingsley Publishers, 2009.

Fellowes, Jessica. "Why Do So Few of Us Know How to Breathe Properly?" *Telegraph*. July 27, 2009. www.telegraph.co.uk/lifestyle/wellbeing/5901075/Why-do-so-few-of-us-know-how-to-breathe-properly.html.

Harvard Health Publishing. "Giving Thanks Can Make You Happier." *Health-beat*. Accessed July 22, 2019. www.health.harvard.edu/healthbeat/giving-thanks-can-make-you-happier.

Harvard Health Publishing. "Stress and the Sensitive Gut." *Harvard Mental Health Letter*. August 2010. www.health.harvard.edu/newsletter_article/stress-and-the-sensitive-gut.

Iowa State University. "More Than Just a Cue, Intrinsic Reward Helps Make Exercise a Habit." ScienceDaily. September 13, 2016. www.sciencedaily.com/releases/2016/09/160913101129.htm.

Lasater, Judith. *Relax and Renew: Restful Yoga for Stressful Times.* Berkeley, CA: Rodmell Press, 1995.

Mayo Clinic. "Back Pain." August 4, 2018. www.mayoclinic.org/diseases-conditions/back-pain/symptoms-causes/syc-20369906.

Mayo Clinic. "Relaxation Techniques: Try These Steps to Reduce Stress." April 19, 2017. www.mayoclinic.org/healthy-lifestyle/stress-management/in-depth/relaxation-technique/art-20045368.

Mental Health America. "Rest, Relaxation, and Exercise." Accessed July 3, 2019. www.mentalhealthamerica.net/conditions/rest-relaxation-and-exercise/.

Tello, Monique. "Regular Meditation More Beneficial Than Vacation." *Harvard Health Blog.* October 27, 2016. www.health.harvard.edu/blog/relaxation-benefits-meditation-stronger-relaxation-benefits-taking-vacation-2016102710532.

Wei, Marlynn. "More Than Just a Game: Yoga for School-Age Children." *Harvard Health Blog.* August 30, 2016. www.health.harvard.edu/blog/more-than-just-a-game-yoga-for-school-age-children-201601299055.

Winerman, Lea. "By the Numbers: Our Stressed-Out Nation." American Psychological Association. December 2017. www.apa.org/monitor/2017/12/numbers.

Woodyard, Catherine. "Exploring the Therapeutic Effects of Yoga and Its Ability to Increase Quality of Life." *International Journal of Yoga* 4, no. 2 (July 2011): 49–54. doi:10.4103/0973-6131.85485.

Yale University. "Stress May Cause Excess Abdominal Fat in Otherwise Slender Women, Study Conducted at Yale Shows." *ScienceDaily.* November 23, 2000. www.sciencedaily.com/releases/2000/11/001120072314.htm.

Index

Acknowledgments

First and foremost, I bow my head in deepest respect to all of my teachers and their teachers, especially Shannon Paige for giving me the (five-star) gift of restorative yoga and encouraging me to share it with others, and Judith Hanson Lasater for pioneering this healing modality.

Mum, I would never be here if you hadn't put me on the path of meditation, yoga, and Ayurveda all those years ago, so, thank you for always knowing what's best.

Thanks to my many guardian angels who have held me above water over the years, especially Cindy Story and Jon Hart. I'd be nowhere without you. Thanks also to my number-one cheerleader, Brian.

Thanks to Sean and the team at Callisto for the opportunity, tremendous organizational support, and belief in my abilities to write this book.

And finally, 108 pranams to the Trinity and all my Mountain Souldiers for holding space while I dove into the writing process.

It was my great pleasure and honor.